42 KM OF RUNLIGION

[S.Kuoan10bulls]

BlueRose ONE.com
Stories Matter
NewDelhi • London

BLUEROSE PUBLISHERS
India | U.K.

BlueRose ONE
Stories Matter
NewDelhi • London

For permissions, requests or inquiries regarding this publication, please contact:

BLUEROSE PUBLISHERS
www.BlueRoseONE.com
info@bluerosepublishers.com
+91 8882 898 898
+4407342408967

ISBN: 978-93-7018-617-0

Cover Design: Shuham Verma
Typesetting: Sagar

First Edition: July 2025

Dedicated

TO

Mr. Milind Soman, and all marathon organizers like PikuSports and all who are engaged in promoting running habit in the world and all following unsung hero of regular walker/runner in Chilla Sports Complex, Delhi, India.

Knowing by name

(1)Mr. Sunder Karki.(2) Mr. Sharad Jain.(3) Ms Suman Jain.(4) Mr Vinod Gupta.(5) Dr. Ashutosh Singh.(6) Mr. S.P.Sharma (7) Mr.Sanjive Bhargava (8) Ms Vijaya Uniyal (9) Mr.Birpal Singh (10) Mr.Rajesh Sharma (11) Mr.G. D. Mishra (12) Mr. Amrendra Mishra (13) Mr. Kuldeep Singh Choudhary (14) Mr. Jagvir Singh (15)Mr. Shive Kumar (16) Mr. Devender Sharma (17) Mr. Jagish Prasad Sharma (18) Mr. Kamal Bhola (19) Mr. Jaman Gotwal (20) Mr.Anuj Gandhi. (21) Mr Mukesh Yadav. (22) Mr. Navendu Prasad (23) Mr. Rajiv Maikhuri. (24) Mr. Ravinder Singh (25)Mr. Vinod Joshi (26)Mr.Surajit Bhattacharjee (27) Mr.Rupanjan Bhattacharjee (28)Mr. Gyanchand (29)Mr. Sankaran (30)Mr. Arun kumar (31)Mr. Biswajit Bhattacharya (32)Mr. Craig Farham (33) Mr. Goodwin (34) Mr.Deepak Bahuguna (35)Mr. Subhash Sharma.(36) Mr.J.P. Sharma (37)Mr J.M. KHAN (38) Mr Naveen Vats (39) Mr. Ratansingh Chauhan.(40) Mr. Ajay Gupta (41) Mr. Bachan Singh Chauhan(42)Mr. Naveen Sharma (43) Mr. Anil Dixit.(44) Mr. Sourabh Chauhan(45) Mr . Subhasish Panda (46) R.M. Pande (47) Mr Anuj Mahto. (48) Mr. Ajay Sriwastaw.(49) Mr. L.B.singh (50)Mr. Rajesh Khanna (51) Mr. Mriganka Ghos.(52) Mr. Prahalad Singh(53) Mr. Atul Mehra (54)Yashpal Chauhan (55)Ms Moutani Goswami (56) Ms Shalini Jain(57) Mr Pranab Mohanty (58) Mr. Manoj Nijhawan.(59) Mr.Gourav Chauhan (60) Mr. P.C. Sharma (61) Mr. Sukhbir Singh Sekhon (62) Mr. Sanjay Kumar Sriwastaw (63) Ms Rajni Varma.(64) Ms Minaxi Arora (65) Ms Manorama Chauhan.(66) Ms. Niru Singhla Sharma (67) Ms Shila Ravi (68) Mr.Rajesh Singh (69) Mr. Rahul Sharma. (70) Abhishek

Chauhan.(71) Pramod Ghate(72)Ms. Mahua Gupta (73) Mr.Namai Das (74) Mr.Umesh Goel (75) Mr. Narendra Mahto. (76) *Maharashtrachi Hasya Jatra.*

And many others not knowing by name.(Unknowingly involved in real great social work- chapter 31 Km)

And my three hearts

Suhani

Sanjali

Sangita.

My mother Late Kuntibai

And Mr. CARLO ROVELL

S.Kuoanıobull

In the world of literature this work may be negligible drop of ocean

But

In the world of runner it may be small cup of drink of motivation.

S.Kuoanıobulls

This book is Beautiful Gift from regular disciplined runners to Non Runners specifically of later age to motivate them for regular walking/running, on the occasion of happy birthday, marriage anniversary and from corporate HR to their employee on any auspicious occasion and New Year.

S.Kuoanıobulls

All thoughts in this book are like various unique flowers in forest because all thought are unedited and completely raw and organic and therefore readers may find it very different and unique natural test during reading of this book and will sense Unique natural fragrance of 42 forest flowers blossomed during 42 days of daily running.

S.Kuoan10bulls

In grammar of every language in the world there are 3 common rules.

1. Letter of alphabet= single entity for single accent =R= Individual boundary. Foundation of any other book and language.

2. Word= Group of letters without gap between them= Run= Combination of letters = Family

3. Sentence= Group of words with gap between them with sense= Society/nation= ***Runligion*** is the Religion of Runners for the runner by the runner to bewilder and enlighten non-runner/walker. Synchronization of words with meaningful sense= Humanity stage=No boundary.

S.Kuoan1obulls

A day without laughter is a day wasted

Charlie Chaplin

A day without Run is a day wasted.

S. Kuoanıobulls

Table Of Contents

Preface

Three Jewels

1.(Empirical approach precedes Sermon = trait of true
Enlightened preacher)

2.(Sermon precedes Action= trait of true Teacher)

3. (Reading precedes Gifting= Meaningful Great social work)

I am an average runner and it has been over 10 years since I am hitting the track every morning before 6 am. Occasionally in group running we used to debate on various topics of social, religious etc. One of my running colleagues Sh. Manoj Agrawal prompted and encouraged me to write the book on running after knowing my consistency of running for ten years to share my experience and thoughts in the world of runners. One another running colleague Sh. Prashant Tandon, journalist also encouraged me to shape my perspective in a book form. Since I have a technical background, writing a book has never been part of my skill set. This book is the result of 10 years' experience of in running and of two habits running and reading as well.

Last but not the least I must thank Mr. Devendra Arora who formed a runners group RunXpress, Delhi India and inspired many like me to make daily running a habit.

Table below is the illustration of participation in marathon events in all over the India.

Sr. No	Date	Name of Marathon/Events	Km	Bib No	Timing
1	27-Sep-15	*3rd Dwarka Half Marathon(Delhi)*	15	641	1:50:50
2	25-Oct-15	*H&H RDA half Marathon(Delhi)*	21.1	385	2:38
3	23-Nov-15	*Airtel Delhi half Marathon(Delhi) 2015*	21.1	10137	2:35:18
4	28-Feb-16	*IDBI Federal Insurance New Delhi Marathon2016*	42.2	10023	5:48:32
5	7/31/2016	*Rotary Rain Run (Goa)*	21.21	131	2:28:50
6	9/11/2016	*4th Dwarka Half Marathon(Delhi)*	21.1	2495	2:14:52
7	10/16/2016	Rishikesh Marathon	25	135	4:43
8	10/23/2016	Millenium City Marathon(Half marathon)	21.1	H084	2:06:09
9	11/20/2016	*Airtel Delhi Half Marathon(Delhi) 2016*	21.1	8652	2:34
10	1/15/2017	Standard Chartered Mumbai Marathon	42.19	5325	6:17:50
11	2/26/2017	*IDBI Federal Insurance New Delhi Marathon2017*	42.2	42765	5;08;58
12	5/14/2017	Mukteswar Marathon	21.1	147	2:46
13	9/10/2017	*5th Dwarka Half Marathon(Delhi)*	21.1	373	2:09
14	11/19/2017	*Airtel Delhi half Marathon(Delhi) 2017*	21.1	1995	2:10
15	12/10/2017	12 Hour Stadium Run in Tyagraj Stadium Delhi(Ultra marathon)	72	1256	12.00
16	1/21/2018	Tata Mumbai Marathon	42.96	651	5:10:00
17	9/16/2018	*6th Dwarka Half Marathon(Delhi)*	21.10	21568	2:06:30
18	9/23/2018	*Pacer in Pinkathon Delhi*	21.28	21003	2:33:00
19	10/21/2018	*Airtel Delhi half Marathon(Delhi) 2018*	21.25	1822	1:57:00
20	1/20/2019	Tata Mumbai Marathon	42.90	2130	5:12:14

21	2/24/2 019	*IDBI Federal Insurance New Delhi Marathon2017*	42. 61	441 63	4:41 :42
22	8/25/2 019	*Nainital Monsoon Mountain Marathon*	23. 00	226 2	3:16 :31
23	28- Sep-19	Riding Event by Audax Club Parisien	10 0	125 93T	6:22 :00
24	10/20/ 2019	*Airtel Delhi half Marathon(Delhi) 2019*	21. 10	381 4	2:10 :00
25	8/2/2 020	NGM NOIDA RIDE	50	LC0 4	3:01
26	23/2/ 2020	*IDBI Federal Insurance New Delhi Marathon2020*	42. 1	451 87	4:58
27	16/10 /2022	Vedanta Delhi half Marathon	21. 1	252 0	2:14 ;21
28	26/02 /2023	Apolo Delhi Marathon	42. 2	451 71	5:47 :23
29	18/12 /2022	*12 Hour Stadium Run in Devi Stadium Gurugram (Ultra marathon)*	73	121 31	12
30	6/8/2 023	Freedom Run Indirapuram	21	210 34	2:19 :17
31	10/9/ 2023	Ladakh Marathon	42	447 3	6;49
32	5/11/ 2023	Rishikesh Marathon	35	352 5	3;52 ;54
33	21/1/ 24	Tata Mumbai Marathon	42	406 9	5:27 :39
34	25/2/ 2024	Apollo Delhi Marathon	42. 43	443 03	5:04 :31
35	9/3/2 024	*12 Hour Night Stadium Run in Jawaharlal Nehru Stadium (Ultra marathon)*	73. 37	120 19	12 hr
36	7/4/2 024	KATRA HALF MARATHON	21	211 29	2:36 :42
37	28/7/ 2024	5TH BRG ANNUAL RUN	10	152 9	1:06 :10
38	2/10/ 2024	APEEJAY RUNATHON 2024	16	160 68	1:43 :58
39	20/10 /2024	Vedanta Delhi Half Marathon	21. 1	562 9	2;15 :40
40	10/11 /2024	Rishikesh Marathon	35	350 62	4:17 ::05
41	15/12 /2024	Tata steel world 25 k Kolkota Marathon	25	348 9	2:41 :18
42	19/01 /2025	Tata Mumbai Marathon	42. 83	254 0	5:22 :46
43	23/02 /2025	Apollo Delhi Marathon	42. 33	463 30	4:51 :46

44	27/4/ 2025	TCS WORLD10K Bangaluru Marathon (PROCAM SLAM achiever 2024-2025)	10	334 58	1:02 :30

As per data available in Strava up to 06/06/2025

Total run	2,566
Total distance in km	24,175
PB 10 KM	49:37:00
PB HALF MARATHON	1:56:06
PB MARATHON	4:38:41

During this period of more than ten years running I have developed 5 USP which helps me immensely to remain consistent runner:-

1. Daily running more than 10 KM
2. Starting time of running before 6 A.M.
3. Every Monday is the NO RUN DAY.
4. Posting of every run in various running wattsup/social group to motivate others.
5. Give the kudos daily to all runners who posted their running activity in various running including the strava group to motivate them for consistency (around 100).

This period of more than 10 years of running brought me near the Enlightenment of Running which is the source of this book. I have conceived the new religion i.e. **Runligion**. Basically I am Electrical engineer and I love the philosophy very much and because of this number of thoughts used to enter in my mind daily during the running, were mixture of Technology and philosophy (***Tecnophilosophy***= Analog of each other). Some time running in group of intellectual and debate during running has also become the part of this new parable.

This figure is the mother of *Postface*

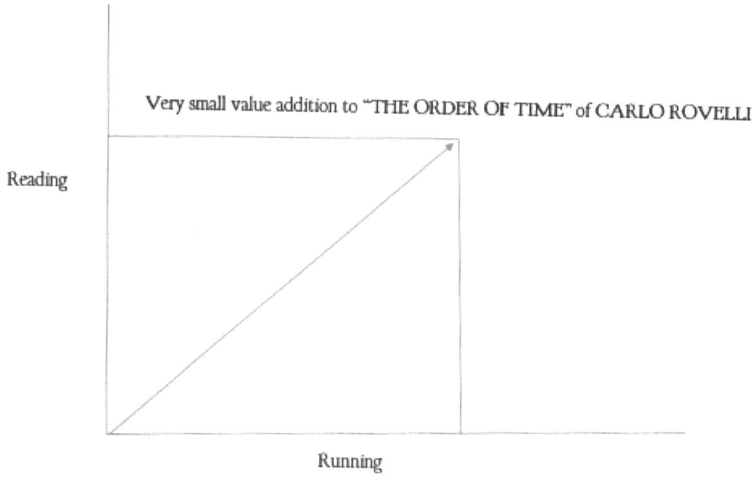

S. Kuoanıobulls

Today's Technophilosophy insight to transform life- Angulimal.

Event name:-Apeejay School NOIDA #RUNATHON2024

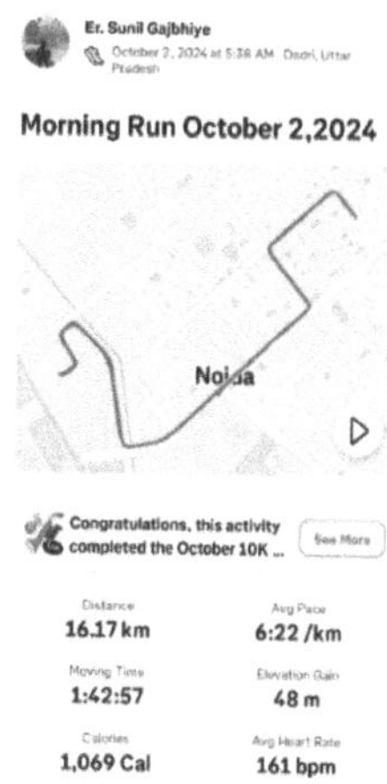

It is often said that when money is lost nothing is lost, when health is lost something is lost and if character is lost everything is lost. In today's world the order of elements of life needs to be changed in the old maxim.

Instead it should be read like this –'when money is lost nothing is lost, when character is lost something is lost and if health is lost everything is lost'. Life we see around teaches us that good health is pivotal for the one's meaningful existence. Money and character can be earned again if health is on your side.

Life is a systematic combination of various energies to experience the existence of world. If you are leading a healthy life only then can you regain the lost money and lost character as well. If you are healthy only then can you become *Angulimal* as per Buddhist scriptures Dhamma or *Balmik* of Ramayan who shunned the evil past and followed the path of dharma. If we consider the soul (*Atma*) as part of God (*Parmatma=Nature=Existence*), then our body is like temple. Keeping very this temple in clean and strong condition must be our prime duty.

Daily running is the cheapest way to stay fit and healthy, best and natural way to keep this real temple of soul clean, strong and in holy condition. Running regularly is like daily worshiping of our won soul for daily resurrection and it develops the courage to explore the new dimension of life and develops extraordinary crises resolving skill. We can keep our sanity intact by running.

1 km

Today's Technophilosophy insight to transform life.

Battery life

What is a healthy life (Technophilosophy)?

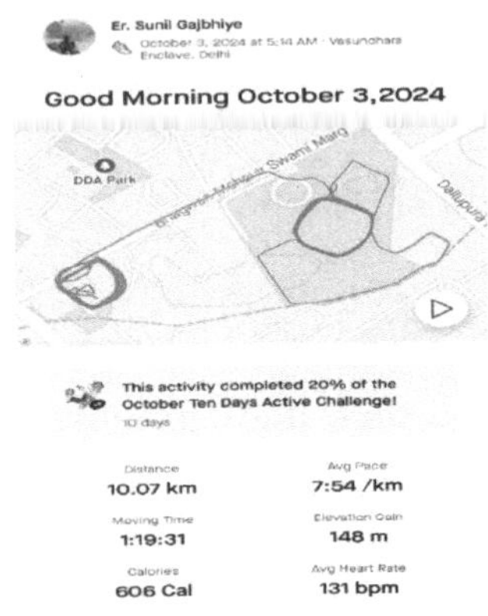
Er. Sunil Gajbhiye
Good Morning October 3,2024
DDA Park
This activity completed 20% of the October Ten Days Active Challenge!
Distance
10.07 km
Avg Pace
7:54 /km
Moving Time
1:19:31
Elevation Gain
148 m
Calories
606 Cal
Avg Heart Rate
131 bpm

Life of a battery can be maximized by equally and timely charging and discharging. In other words battery lives longer if on continuous use and upkeep.

Same principle is applicable to our body.

Charging your body is having healthy food timely every day – when you run a good distance discharging takes place. Key here is the consistency of the timely run daily. Balance between charging and discharging is the universal principle to maintain any system healthy and fruitful. Excess unbalancing between charging and discharging is the rout cause of several physical diseases and mental disorders. Bolt of gold of substandard size is useless in mechanical Engineering. Similarly talents of substandard ethics is not only useless but also most dangerous for the humanity.

Daily disciplined Running is journey from substandard to standard state.

2 km

Today's Technophilosophy insight to transform life

Potential of seed

Every seed has capacity to become tree, only matter is, it needs little courage to stay beneath the soil till sprouting. Likewise every person has the capacity to become runner, only matter is to stay under the soil of discipline till sprouting. Once we achieve the state of sprout, nature itself will take care of journey from "fighting attitude" to "let go attitude" till the first milestone of any new runner.

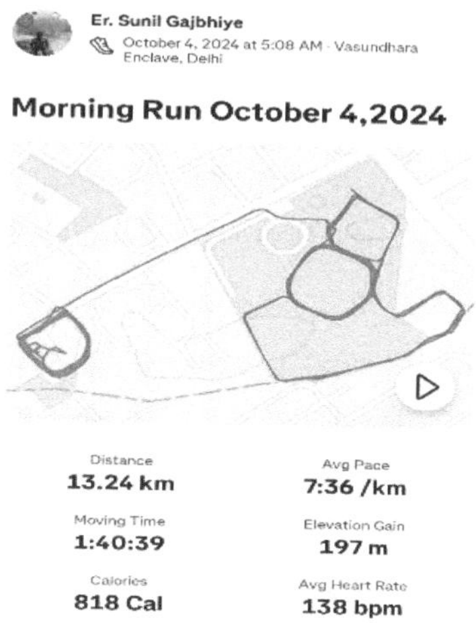
Er. Sunil Gajbhiye
October 4, 2024 at 5:08 AM · Vasundhara Enclave, Delhi
Morning Run October 4,2024
Distance
13.24 km
Avg Pace
7:36 /km
Moving Time
1:40:39
Elevation Gain
197 m
Calories
818 Cal
Avg Heart Rate
138 bpm

Daily regular disciplined running is the only way to attain the state of let-go. Fighting attitude is the part of competition which is the requirement of ego while let-go attitude with awareness is the part of contribution which is the requirement of nature. Competition attitude will lead towards personal development while contribution attitude will lead towards humanity development. Running is the way to create contribution attitude.

First Gear

Starting torque:-Leaving the bed before 6 AM daily is the most difficult task for any new runner and if he succeeded even for one month, the victory of the half battle would be in his bag. This is the first gear of mind. (First month activity).

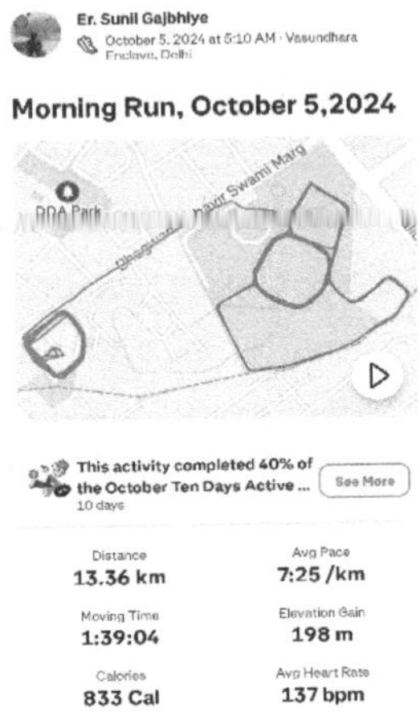

Starting torque is proportional to age of starting Run. Starting at the early age means starting torque will be lower. Hear starting torque is the mechanical word which is analog of MENTAL retardation. For example:-

At the age of 25 years MENTAL BLOCK= 25 Kg

At the age of 50 years MENTAL BLOCK=50 Kg.

For me Starting TORQUE was 55 Kg. because I started running at the age of 55 years.

Therefore "early to bed, early to rise makes man healthy, wealthy and wise" is also very apt maxim for runners. Irrespective of any weight of mental block, all can be removed scientifically gradually at any age of life. According to me consistent daily running is the best physician of mental retardation. Exclusion of comfort zone in morning is conducive to good health and helps to regain lost natural beauty and agility.

Second Gear

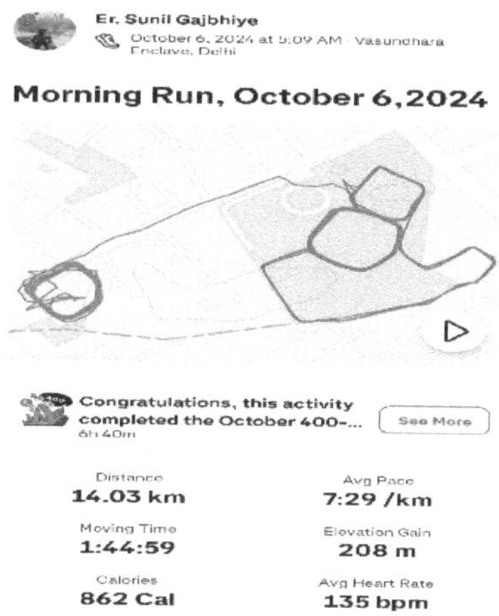
Er. Sunil Gajbhiye
October 6, 2024 at 5:09 AM · Vasundhara Enclave, Delhi
Morning Run, October 6,2024
Congratulations, this activity completed the October 400-...
6h 40m
See More
Distance
14.03 km
Avg Pace
7:29 /km
Moving Time
1:44:59
Elevation Gain
208 m
Calories
862 Cal
Avg Heart Rate
135 bpm

Walking 2 KM alternate day for next one month was the second gear of my mind. (Second month activity). This period is very crucial because mental retardation may be heavy and which may cause failure in this holy scarification.

Our schools are real farms to produce future crops of disciplined good citizens for our nation and this book may be fruitful in this direction if we inculcate the theme of this book on Running and consider this book a passage for future ethically strong nation. Daily running in itself is a unique lesson to learn different state of mind in different time zone and places and is also unique method to enhance endurance of mind. Plants thrive in fertilized soil similarly nation thrive in soil of country having maximum citizens of daily disciplined running habit.

Monday (October 7, 2024) is rest day

5 km

Third Gear

Walking 2 Km daily for one month (six days in a week) was the third gear of my mind (Third month activity). In this period, body starts gaining beautiful momentum and become slowly and gradually part of rejoicing state. In this duration I started to love my whole body and started to measure my own potential and thus automatically entered the new college of MBA i.e.

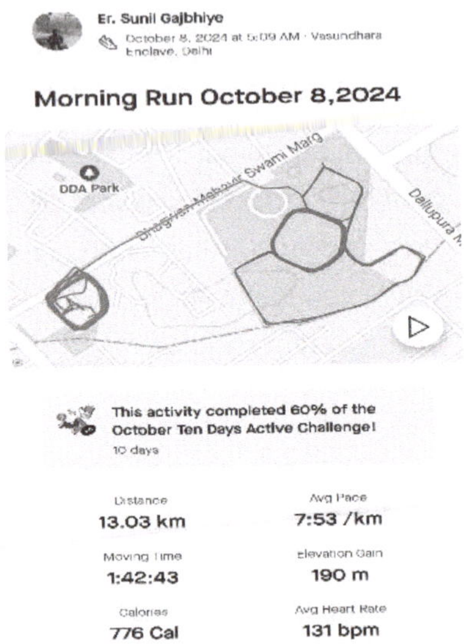

MEASURMENT/MANAGEMENT OF BODY ABILITY .Running teaches us how to be oneself, how to be original and authentic in this world of imitators and this disciplined daily running is precious gift of life. Daily Disciplined Running also teaches us to enjoy ascetic disciplines and not to regress under any adverse condition.

This run is dedicated to Sir Rattan Tata

Walking 1 Km and running 1Km in alternate day (Six days in a week) for one month was the fourth gear of my mind. (Fourth month activity)

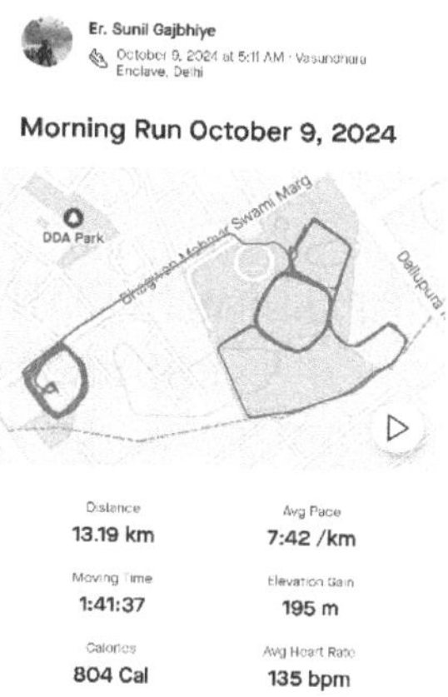
Er. Sunil Gajbhiye
October 9, 2024 at 5:11 AM · Vasundhara Enclave, Delhi
Morning Run October 9, 2024
DDA Park
Swami Marg
Distance
13.19 km
Avg Pace
7:42 /km
Moving Time
1:41:37
Elevation Gain
195 m
Calories
804 Cal
Avg Heart Rate
135 bpm

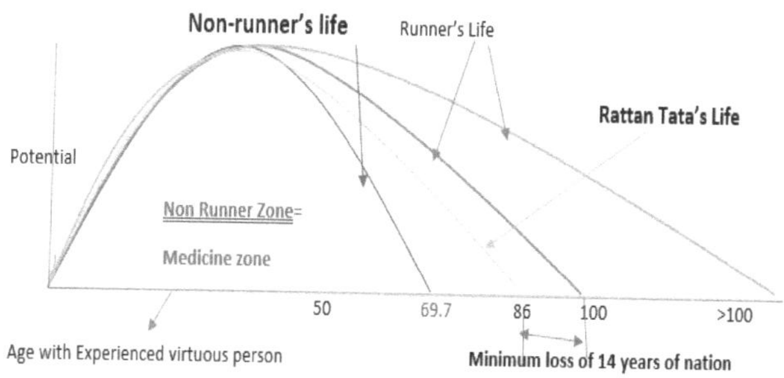

Today's Technophilosophy insight to transform life

Old experienced of virtuous professional, leaders, social workers are the gold for the Nation. All ethical professional, Leader, social worker must run consistently as they are real Gold for nation. If they maximize span of life by running, the nation can extract more valuable contribution from them. According to me, today such loss of minimum 14 years of our nation has been occurred because of demise of Shree Ratan Tata sir, as he died at the age of 86 years (100-86=14).(*The average life expectancy in India in 2022 was 69.7 years below global average 72.6)*

Top Gear

Running more than 3 Km daily (Six days in a week) was the top gear of my mind to attain the proper momentum. (Fifth month activity).

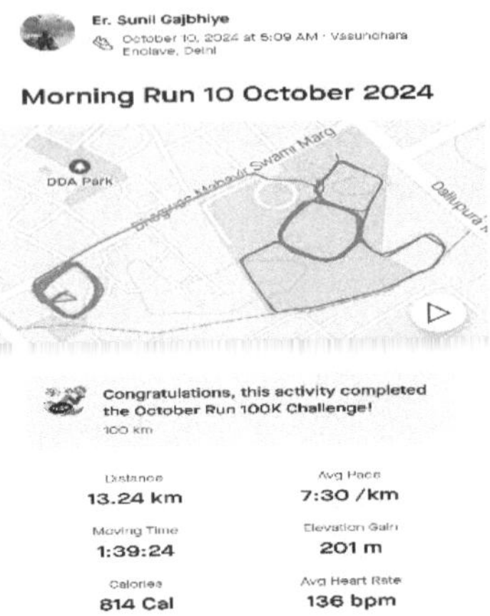
Er. Sunil Gajbhiye
October 10, 2024 at 5:09 AM · Vasundhara Enclave, Delhi
Morning Run 10 October 2024
DDA Park
Congratulations, this activity completed the October Run 100K Challenge!
100 km
Distance
13.24 km
Avg Pace
7:30 /km
Moving Time
1:39:24
Elevation Gain
201 m
Calories
814 Cal
Avg Heart Rate
136 bpm

MEASURMENT/MANAGEMENT OF BODY ABILITY.

By this time mental momentum has been attained and mind started to enjoy the running because of resurrection of personality with each run. It was like birth trouble for me. I have given the birth to new child inside my own personality having the trait of running right from this birth. Birth trouble before the birth of this running child, gave me immense happiness after the birth of this running child inside my mind. Now taking the care of this running child has become holy duty of mother mind inside me and this holy duty is the source of all kind of happiness in this world for me. This feeling of happiness of motherhood helps me to enjoy the daily running and thus enter the virtuous cycle (discipline) from vicious cycle (indiscipline).

Virtuous cycle= Daily discipline running.

Vicious cycle= No run or rare run

Blissful dance of inner being

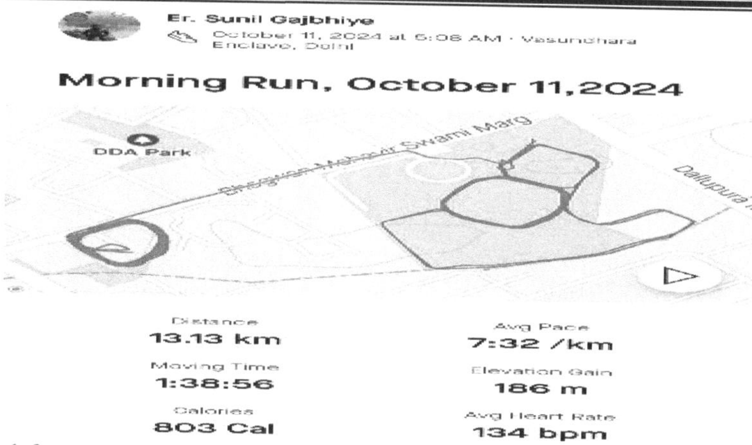

Fuel for next day running:-After achieving the target of running of more than 10 Km daily, I feel the blissful dance of inner being daily and feel like king of my own world after running more than 10 km and preserve it for next day running which made me consistent runner. To remain in the area of virtuous cycle forever, the feeling of inexpressible inner blissfulness must be part of daily running. In electrical lamp-

Power (converted into light) $=I^{2}XR$

Here I=current, R= Resistance of filament

Power of Inexpressible inner blissfulness (inner light) $= D^{2}x\ R$

Here D= distance covered in running,

R= resistance of Vicious cycle (laziness) to be overcome.

As per ***technophilosophy*** daily disciplined running will beget daily blissfulness which will be root cause of consistent running. To become the real runner one must leave aside ephemeral comfort zone for lasting happiness and for this one must comprehend the trick of mind who always tries to keep you in futile comfort zone.

9 km

Vicious and virtuous cycle

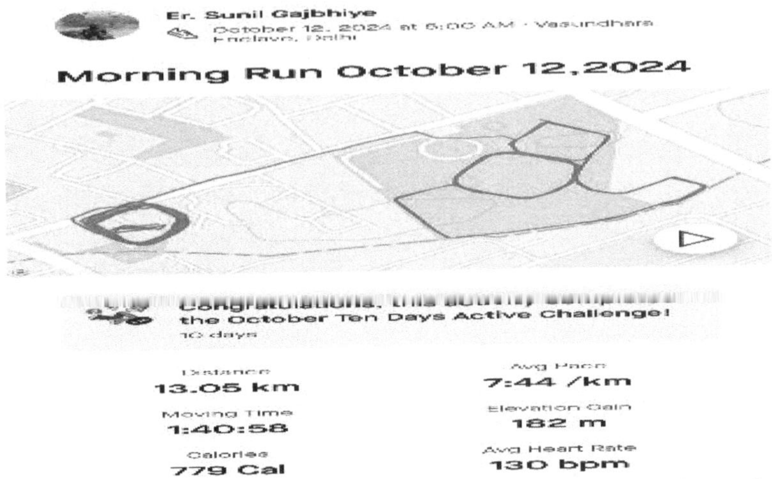

Now keep your foot on escalators to reach mile stone of 5 km, 10km, 15 km, half marathon and marathon. Many small time bound targets are sources of great success. After reaching every mile stone, preserve test of success for next mile stone. This preserved test will propel you for daily running

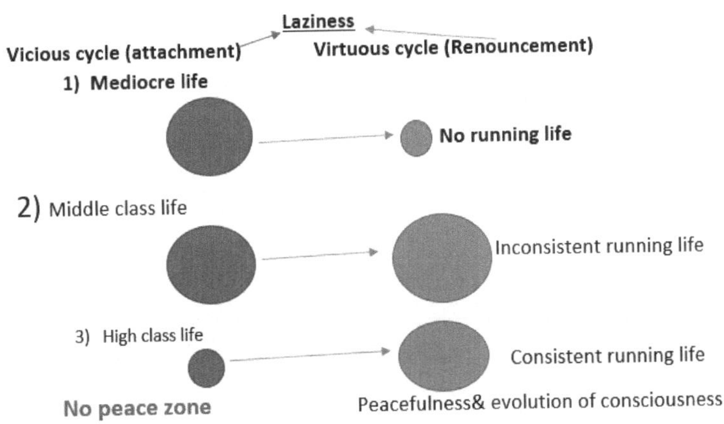

Escape Velocity

Why only running? Today's technophilosophy thought during running

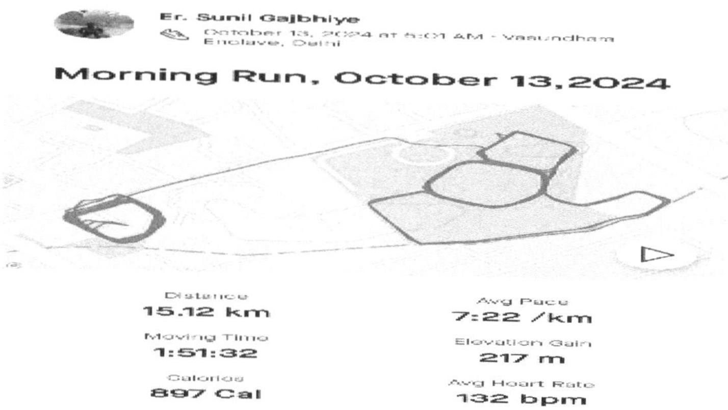

Running is the natural exercise. Look at the birds, in the morning most of them run in sky in form of flying. If we observe the activities of all animal, all of them do this natural exercise. Natural movement is the symbol of life and during running all inner and outer limbs of the body along with the soul become the part of running which is very much essential for healthy body.

Top gear of running is like gaining the escape velocity, which is capable to cross the gravitational area of earth. Here gravitational area is our tendency to be in harmful comfortable zone and once we overcome it we can become like satellite which revolve around the earth in specific orbit with discipline. This state facilitates the consistency in running behavior like satellites consistent movement, which is very much essential for Self-Actualization (Top need of Maslow's Hierarchy of five needs)

Monday (October 14, 2024) is rest day.

11 km

Well of fresh water

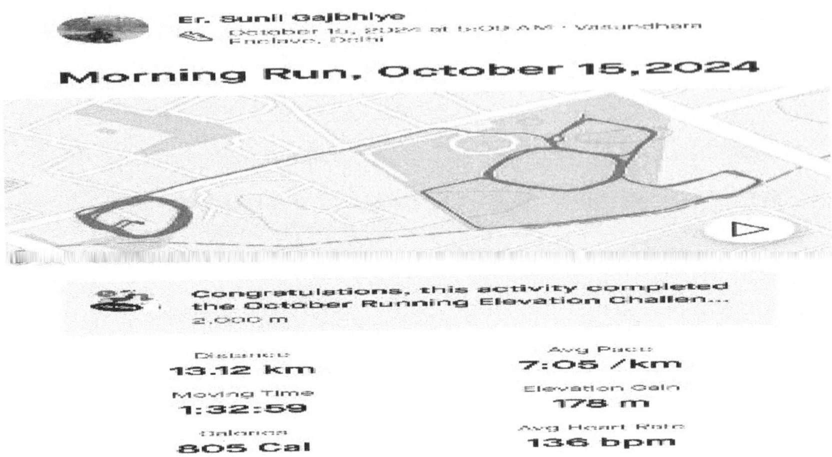

Running convert body into well of fresh water. If we don't take out the water from well daily, its water become stinking, no potable after some time because of scientific reason. If we don't take water from well regularly, the level of water inside the well will increase and this will increase the pressure on the hole of incoming water from nature and it will close the sources of fresh water eventually. And after some time it becomes noisome, stale because of no incoming fresh water from nature. Sweating during running is like taking water from the well of your body to maintain the healthiness and it is also equal to nourishment, as accumulated harmful element in body because of contaminated foods and poor air quality, gets way to leave the body through sweating which play role of natural antidote. After inculcating this theory of well of fresh water we can maintain the perpetuation state of running in contaminated atmosphere and that is what existence wants us to do. Thus daily running is the device to tune with nature.

12 km

Value of fast

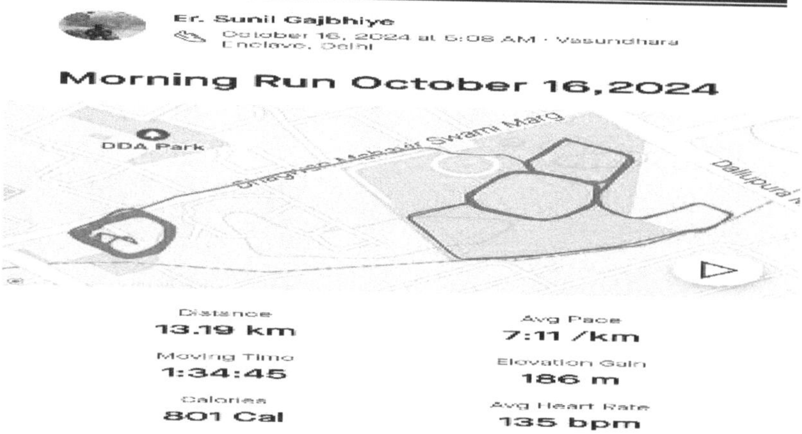

As I have to participated in Vedanta Delhi Half marathon on October 20, 2024, I am going to take break of 3 days from 17 to 19 October as per my own rule of ***Runligion***. This is also the part of my discipline of running. This break is nothing but one kind of fast of running for me. I will have breakfast of 21 km on October 20, 2024. Breaking of fast is breakfast. Fast is real spices of food. Eating food without appetite is also burden on the body. Daily running helps me to stimulate appetite daily and thus makes my meal real natural delicious daily. Feeding the body with joy is spiritual procedure to me and this is possible only after the proper break of fast. Running precedes fast and fast precedes Breakfast like cause precedes effect. Sidharth Goutam was also enlightened and became Buddha only after very long fast as per *Buddhist* scripture. When Sidharth determined not to give up mediation stage before attaining the Enlightenment, after very long period of fast, when he became emaciated and the part of Banyan tree under which he was meditating, ate rice pudding offered by Sujata, wife of farmer and then within short period of further meditation he attained **Enlightenment** and became **Buddha**. So proper and adequate fast is catalyst agent to achieve calm and quite state of mind after breakfast.

13 km

Fast, breakfast and festival

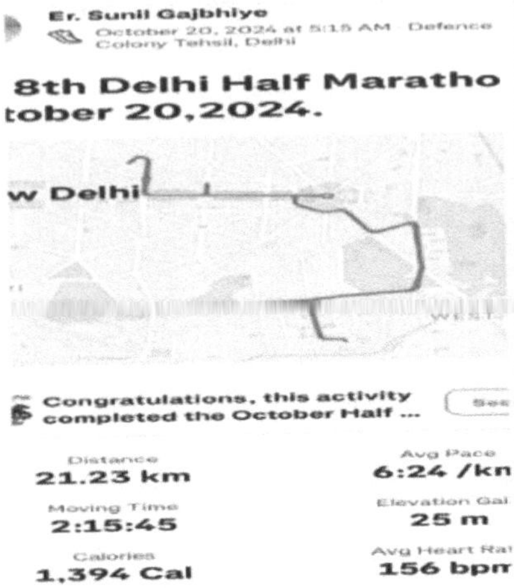
Er. Sunil Gajbhiye
October 20, 2024 at 5:15 AM · Defence Colony Tehsil, Delhi
8th Delhi Half Maratho
tober 20,2024.
w Delhi
Congratulations, this activity completed the October Half ...
Distance
21.23 km
Avg Pace
6:24 /kn
Moving Time
2:15:45
Elevation Gai
25 m
Calories
1,394 Cal
Avg Heart Ra
156 bpn

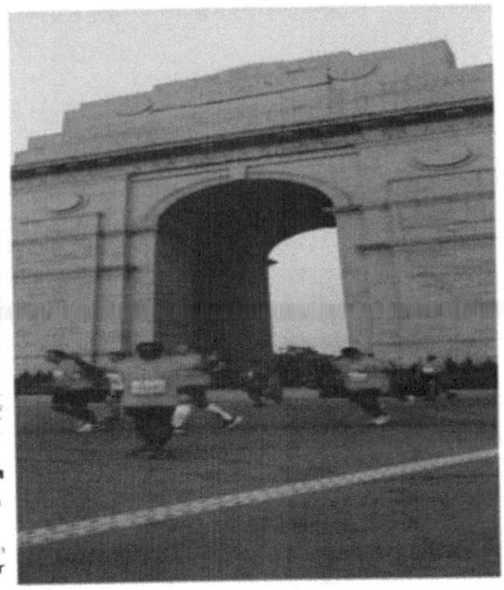

After the fast of 3 days today I have participated in Vedanta Delhi Half Marathon with around 36000 runners and it was delicious and delighted breakfast to me. After touching the finishing line I felt blissful dance of my soul and which was celebration of festival for me. It is true festival of humanity because this is the only festival which is celebrated by all human being irrespective of their religion, cast, creed and nation. The enthusiasm of participant was nothing but way to Fit Humanity Movement after freedom movement. This is the only festival of human being where we can learn and understand the value of peace and serenity. This notion helps to inculcate to make running behavior as part of our daily activity and provides strong enthusiasm for another upcoming marathon and become the part of virtuous cycle.

Monday (October 21, 2024) is rest day

14 km

Health Budget & Running

Running must be part of course right from 1st class to achieve the goal of Fit India as a long term planning. Short term gain is the source of long term pain and long term prudent plan is source of long lasting permanent gain.

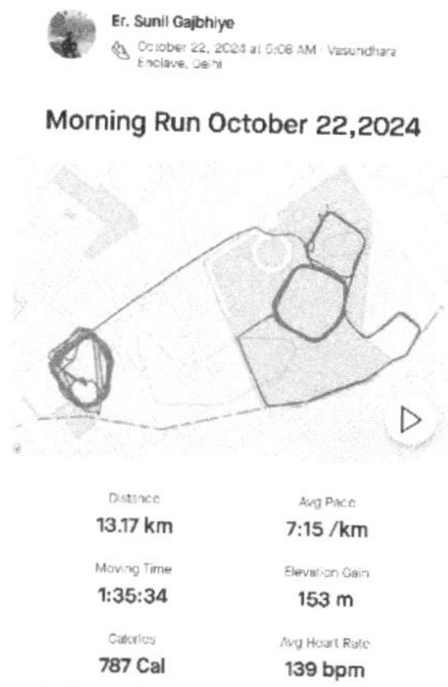
Er. Sunil Gajbhiye
Morning Run October 22,2024
Distance
13.17 km
Avg Pace
7:15 /km
Moving Time
1:35:34
Elevation Gain
153 m
Calories
787 Cal
Avg Heart Rate
139 bpm

Budget(24-25) of India	In crore	Percentage
Health (12.9% increase)	90958.63	96.3535113
sport	3442.32	3.64648873
Health +sport	94400.95	100
Running (20%)	18880.19	

From above chart if our government allocate 20 % of Health and sport budget to only running activity in India it may fetch 80 % good result in form of Healthy Fit India. According to me increasing in health budget every year is nothing but is indication of poor awareness of people toward the health. In 80% cases of health problem, public is responsible due to their negligence attitude towards their own health. So running awareness program can be very fruitful and prudent step for development of developing country like India. For "dignity of individual" health awareness of individual is most important gradient which is the foundation of fraternity to build the strong nation. Daily running habit of citizens is the best way to begat fraternity. Formula for healthy nation:-

Increasing of number of runners in country will cause significant reduction in health budget in future, which is essential gradient for strong and healthy nation.

15 km

Comfort vs Endurance

You must be the doctor of your own body during the running. Never unheard (ignore) the language of pain. Always treat it as the patient. "No pain No gain" is true but "excess of everything is poison" is also equally true. Therefore endurance to bear the pain should be gradual and then only will it graduate you as a successful finisher marathoner. It should be like string of *Vina*. To get the melodious music from VINA we need to tight the string very carefully till before the breaking point of string.

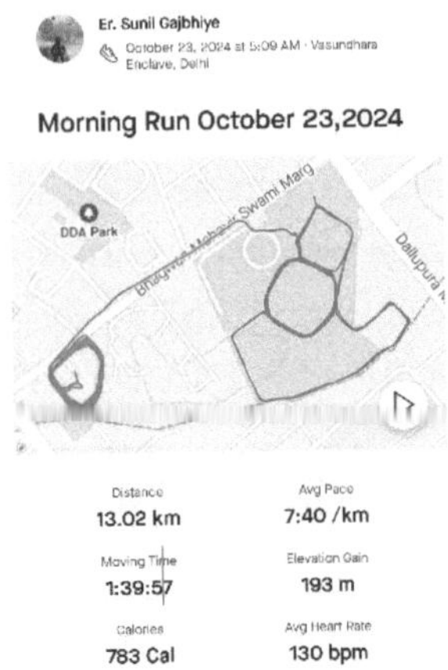

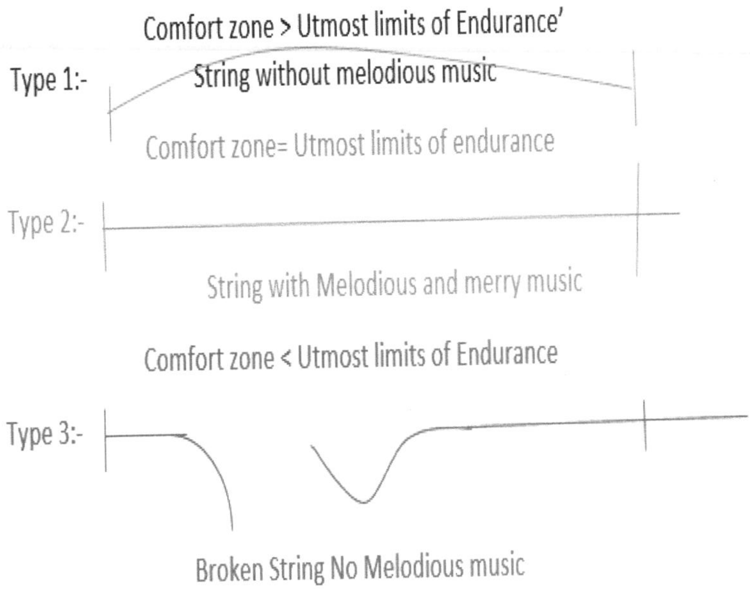

16 km

Might is Right VS Right is Might which is the real art of life.

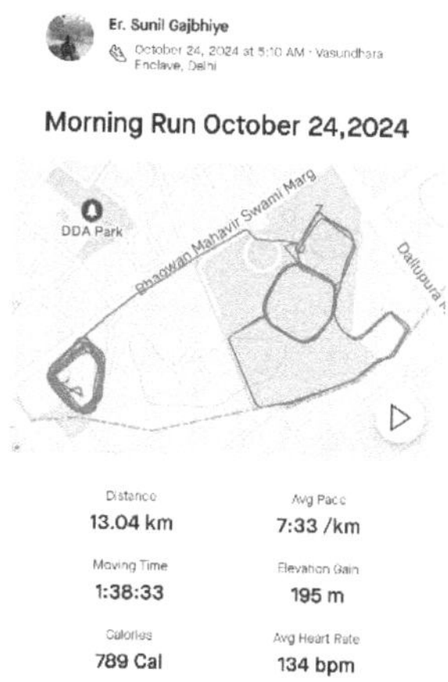

Er. Sunil Gajbhiye
October 24, 2024 at 5:10 AM · Vasundhara Enclave, Delhi
Morning Run October 24,2024
DDA Park
Bhagwan Mahavir Swami Marg
Distance
13.04 km
Avg Pace
7:33 /km
Moving Time
1:38:33
Elevation Gain
195 m
Calories
789 Cal
Avg Heart Rate
134 bpm

Might is right is the old famous proverb which is suitable to only undemocratic and dictatorship countries. As per this saying only person having the power can be enjoyed their life. ***(Jiski Lathi uski Bhaish ,Jungal raj in Hindi)***

Transformation of old proverb into Maxim is symbol of progress.

"Right (Running) is Might" is maxim against old proverb. Running provides healthy body, symbol of might. Healthy body is abode of healthy mind which is inevitable part for development, progress for any developing country like India because only healthy peaceful mind consider humanity as part of progress. Sick mind with power (Might) is the source of various ill acts which is against the Devine humanity. Daily running is the real catalyst for deep calmness which is abode of valued humanity to experience transcendence. Daily running is also journey from agony to ecstasy means journey from "Might is Right" to "Right is Might"

This is absolute immobile insight state. To me daily running is creative art to achieve the consistency because running is the scale of self-potential which helps to reach near the culmination of joy of "Right is Might" which is the magnificence of running.

Satyamev Jayte ("सत्यमेव जयते") = Right is Might= Foundation of Indian democracy.

17 km

Light and Delight

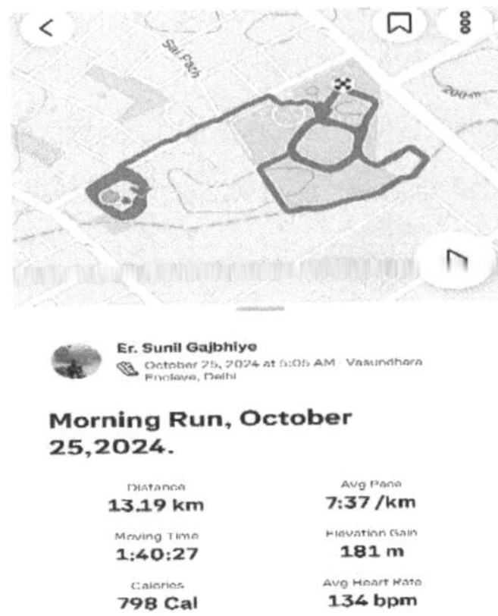
Er. Sunil Gajbhiye
October 25, 2024 at 5:05 AM · Vasundhara Enclave, Delhi
Morning Run, October 25,2024.
Distance
13.19 km
Avg Pace
7:37 /km
Moving Time
1:40:27
Elevation Gain
181 m
Calories
798 Cal
Avg Heart Rate
134 bpm

Light and delight. What is the light? Light is the result of flame burning of candle which killed darkness around it. It means light is absent of darkness. In the same way Running is the burning process which generate the awareness which is the absent of ego. It means running helps me to reduce the amount of ego gradually to attained serenity and delight eventually. **Physical running activity releases endorphins, serotonin, and dopamine, which can contribute to feelings of delight and euphoria.** This delight helps to develop awareness.

Awareness helps to keep misery away.

Pilgrimage of daily running--

Uncompassionate →

Running addiction →

Delight-→

Awareness- →

Prosperity→

Compassionate

Will be out of Delhi from October 26 to 31 .2024

18 km

Power factor

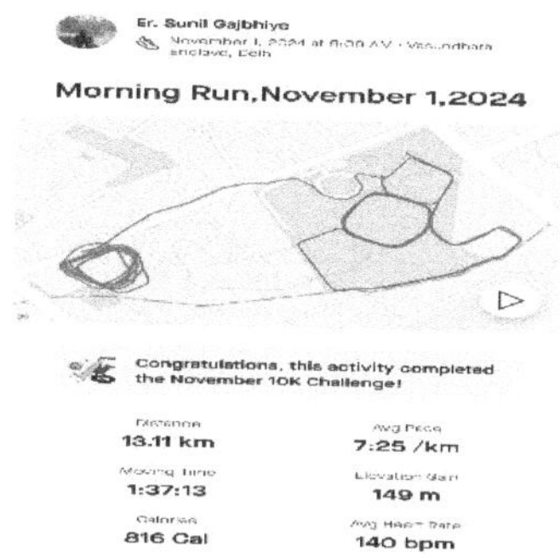

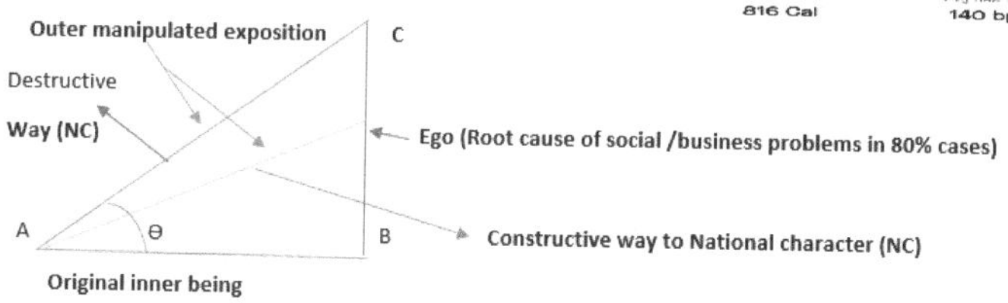

Cos Θ=Power factor= Scale of National character as per my *Technophilosophy*

If Θ=0 Then Cos (0) =1 (Trait of saint =state of tranquility)

Original inner being = Outer exposition (No double face state)

Cos (0) x 100=1x100=100=Tranquility state

When there is no outer manipulated exhibition then it provides the place of trust amongst various parties. Trust is the bottom line of success for any kind of social business.

If Θ=90 then Cos (90) =0 (Trait of devil=state of anxiety).All applied effort will have zero result for nation.

Cos (90) x100= 0x100=0=Restless state

Mistrust is the biggest obstacle for any social business

Running has helped me to reduce the *EGO* and improved the power factor of my personality.

Improved tranquility always helps in critical situation of life to overcome it.

Resident of disciplined home

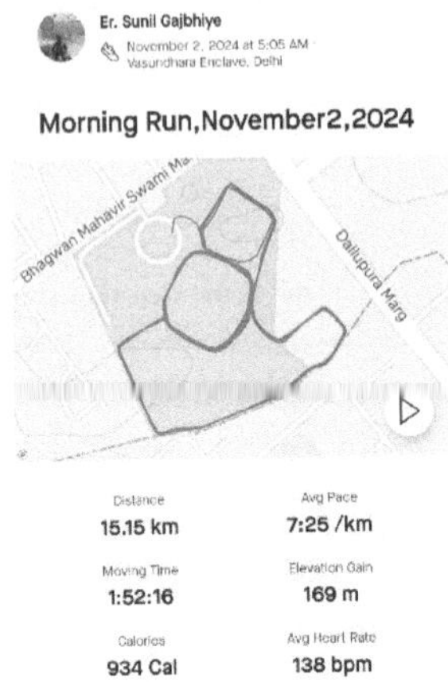

For most of people, discipline is most dangerous word in their life and that is why they never become the disciple of discipline. But regular running teaches how to enjoy the discipline which is very helpful in any other constructive work of life.

Potential energy= mgh, m=mass, g=gravitational force (comfort zone), h=height

Kinetic Energy=1/2 mv^2, m=mass, v= velocity

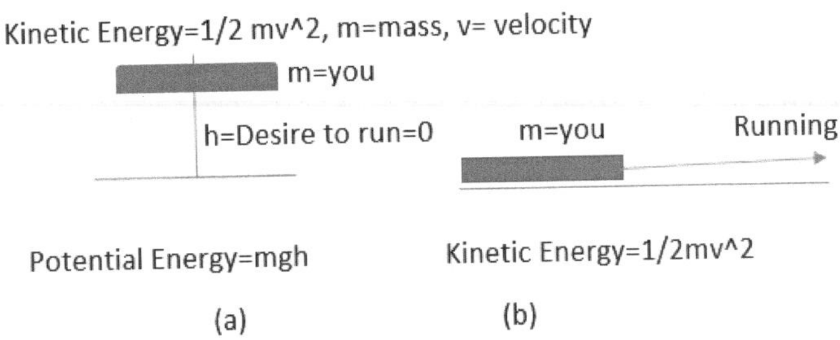

Picture (a) is illustration of unused energy in the body which will allow enemy of body to play their role to invite various dieses in future. Picture (b) is illustration of utilization of energy which prevents the enemy of body to play their role to invite various dieses and keeps u healthy and makes you resident of disciplined home. Transformation of PE into KE leads towards tranquility because during running there is movement of all inner part of body which keeps you far away from hospital. Hospital is symbol of two type of losses, first economic losses and second is peace of mind losses of whole family concerned which is invaluable. Thus daily disciplined running provides daily moment of glory.

Journey of Democracy from childhood to Maturity stage.

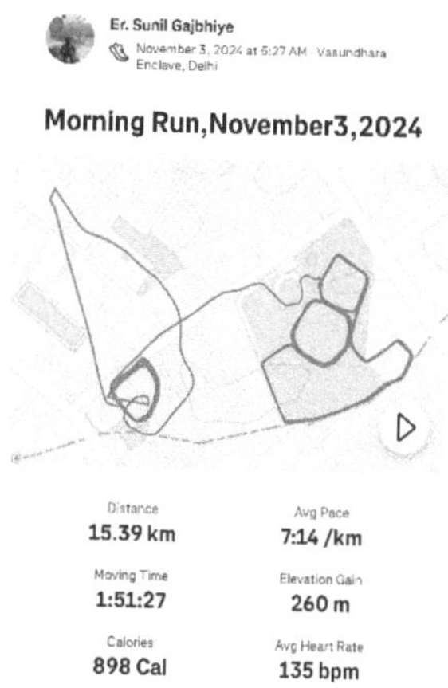

Er. Sunil Gajbhiye
November 3, 2024 at 5:27 AM · Vasundhara Enclave, Delhi
Morning Run,November3,2024
Distance
15.39 km
Avg Pace
7:14 /km
Moving Time
1:51:27
Elevation Gain
260 m
Calories
898 Cal
Avg Heart Rate
135 bpm

Age of American democracy from 1630 to 2024 is 394 years. Date of Woman right to vote in America is June 4, 1919 after 289 years after birth of Democracy. It means unhealthy democracy was in America for almost 280 years. And it took 280 years to become near mature democracy. Because keeping woman out of democracy process right from beginning in itself is birth of unhealthy child (democracy). Age of Indian Democracy from 26 Jan 1950 to 26 Jan 2024 is 76 years with equal voting right to man and woman and thus Indian baby democracy is healthier than USA baby democracy from voting point of view at the time of its birth. If we consider our democracy as baby democracy then it is our duty to take the proper care of it first, from health point of view. During learning of walking, baby falls so many times. So falling and rising is the part of childhood and it's applicable to baby democracy as well. As per nature law every baby needs some period to become mature, subject to its health condition. Shortening the immaturity period of democracy is possible if we take proper and prudent steps right from its childhood by making running compulsory course for student right from first standard in school. For example for class 1, daily 100 meters, for class 2, daily 200 meters,---for class 10,daily 1 km so on-- The fruit of this prudent step for the nation will be visible after at least 20 years. This is the only process to beget future good citizens.

Monday (November 4, 2024) is rest day

21 km

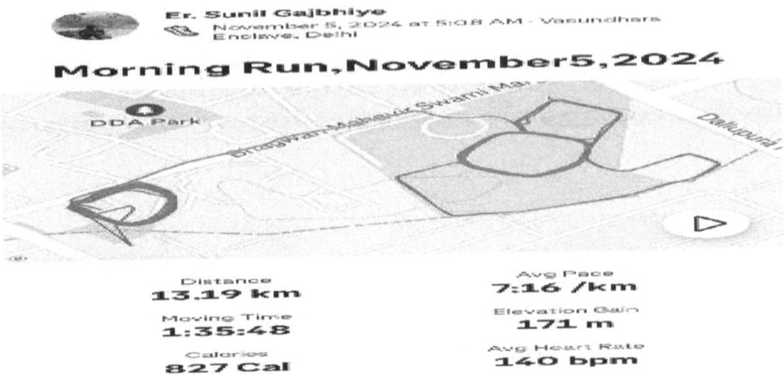

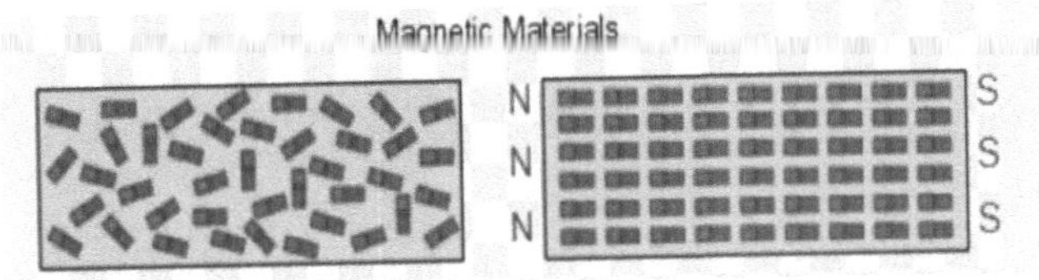

(A) Country of no runner with diversity (B) Nation of Runligion.

Democracy is the system to convert country (house) into Nation (home), like Magnetization is the process to convert nonmagnetic iron into magnet. Country is the boundary while nation is the quality of cordial relation among citizens within boundary. In the magnet all molecules are in straight line (B) that's why it has the power to attract the simple iron, it means all of them are part of discipline while in nonmagnetic iron, all its molecules are not in straight line (A) it means all of them are part of indiscipline and hence zero power of magnetic attraction . Country like India having numbers of religions, caste, creed, and languages are of type (A) country means unity in diversity which is only metaphor in philosophy books and in lectures but in pragmatic it becomes very difficult to convert it into Nation. Nonmagnetic iron become the magnate after fixed considerable period of staying in the magnetic field. Participation of maximum people of the country in daily running activity will transform the country (Nonmagnetic Iron) into nation (Magnet) and which will be conducive to reach the Road to True Nation. Propagation of *Runligion* at this juncture to obtain the utopian democracy is very important because even today it is the childhood stage of our democracy from history point of view.

Opposite pole

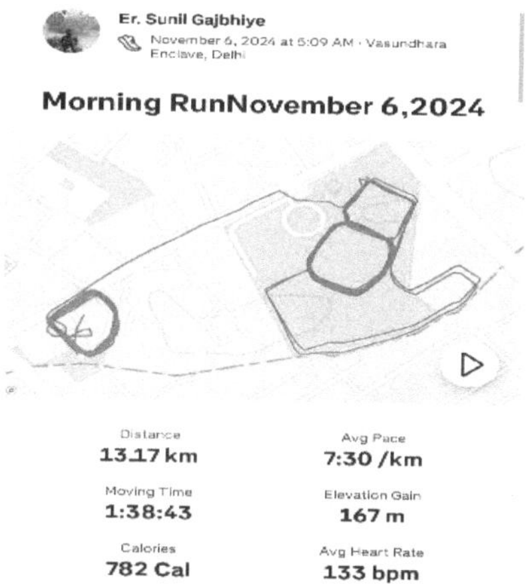
Er. Sunil Gajbhiye
November 6, 2024 at 5:09 AM · Vasundhara Enclave, Delhi
Morning RunNovember 6,2024
Distance
13.17 km
Avg Pace
7:30 /km
Moving Time
1:38:43
Elevation Gain
167 m
Calories
782 Cal
Avg Heart Rate
133 bpm

The magnet has two poles, North Pole and South Pole. Unlike poles attract each other as North Pole attracts South Pole of another magnet and like poles repeal each other as North Pole repeals North Pole of another magnet. Similarly short term pain of daily running attracts the long term gain in day to day life in form of healthy body. If you know the period of pain which is possible in running activity, then it is not the pain but source of amusement. This notion will create the enjoyment of

The short term pain of running daily.

Will attract the long term happiness surely.

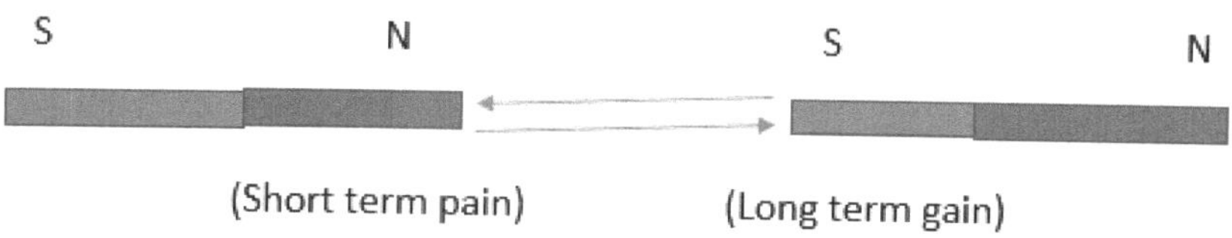

As, I have to participated in Rishikesh marathon (35Km) on November 10, 2024,I am going to take break of 5 days from November 7, 2024 to November 11,2024. This is also the part of my discipline of running. Running to me is a spiritual phenomenon.

23 km

Spiritual Running in hilly terrain on the bank of Ganga River.

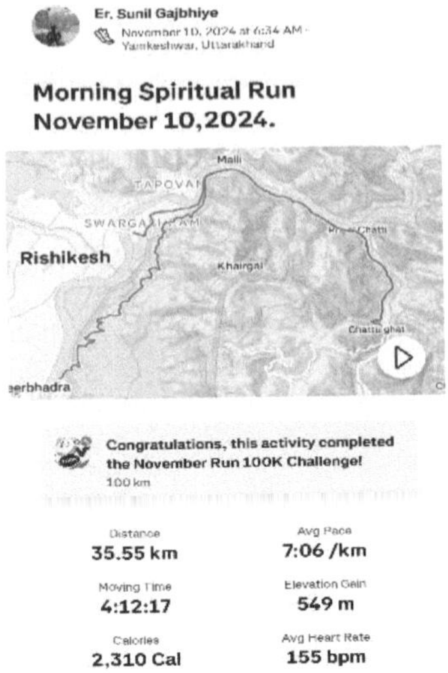

During activity of marathon of 35 Km in Rishikesh, after 15 Km when I was ***alone*** in deep forest, I found myself completely at the lap of Nature. This running was unique type of meditation for me.

Spiritual=*Adhyatm*= *Adhyan+Atma* (***आत्मा का अध्ययन)***=Self Study of soul→Path toward-> Swadhinta (स्वाधीनता)=Swayam Ke Adhin Hona = self-control of Mind=>Freedom of soul from garbage like hate, jealousy etc.=>create the place in mind for peace. During period of 4:12:17, I found myself in the area of true Aloneness of whole =All in One= real complete blissful stage=virus free stage of mind. Mind became abode of whole nature and I became the part Nature it means disappearance of sense of *Loneliness*= Less in one= Temporal desires= Mind with various virus like jealousy, hate etc. Real Cloud before me was mirror of cloud of my mind like phantasmagoria because of which I was far away from truth of blissful stage of mind. Momentary transformation of consciousness from ego to egoless state was beautiful experience for me. During running I found third state of Mind –

1st Unconsciousness---abode of very powerful sinner, contains 80% past

2nd Consciousness--abode of saint, generally very weak, contains 20% present.

3rd Super consciousness -abode of unbiased Judge during conflict between sinner and saint.

Monday (November 11, 2024) is rest day

24 km

When running becomes part of your blood, bones and marrow then you enter into the real paradise of your life only very in this earth and consistent running will enchant you daily. If gap without solid reason creates the guilt in you then you consider yourself as follower of **Runlegion** because that very guilt becomes the driving force to rise and run again next morning.

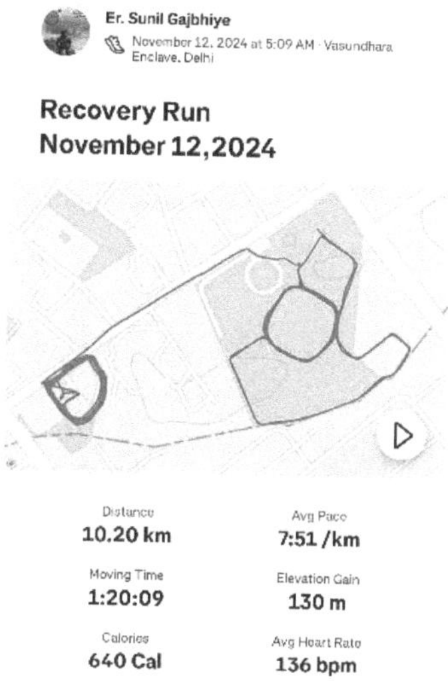
Er. Sunil Gajbhiye
November 12, 2024 at 5:09 AM · Vasundhara Enclave, Delhi
Recovery Run
November 12,2024
Distance
10.20 km
Avg Pace
7:51 /km
Moving Time
1:20:09
Elevation Gain
130 m
Calories
640 Cal
Avg Heart Rate
136 bpm

As per my Technophilosophy:-

In Hindi Safal (सफल) means success.

In English also fruition means success. In both language success is related to delicious fruits.

स -> स्वादिस्ट -> **फल**= **सफल**

(Delicious fruits for others not for tree itself which produces, means helping others without expectation).

Expectation is source of disappointment and disappointment is source of grief.

Tree begets the delicious fruits for others not for itself, therefore, it is the real success of tree. Daily discipline running and its positing in social media to motivate non-runners is the process to beget fruits for others like tree. All runners have the inner inexpressible blissful state of mind and expressing it to others to motivate them as sharing is the real social works and it is real success if you motivate others to run daily. So all marathon organizers are doing real social work and helping for building the strong nation because all of them are engaged in this holy cause.

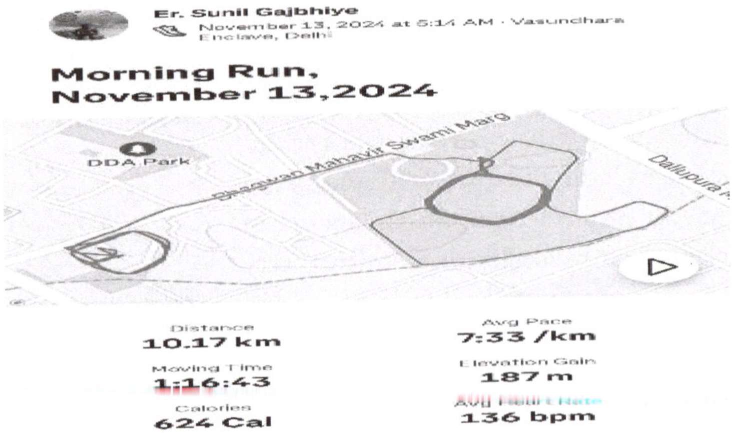

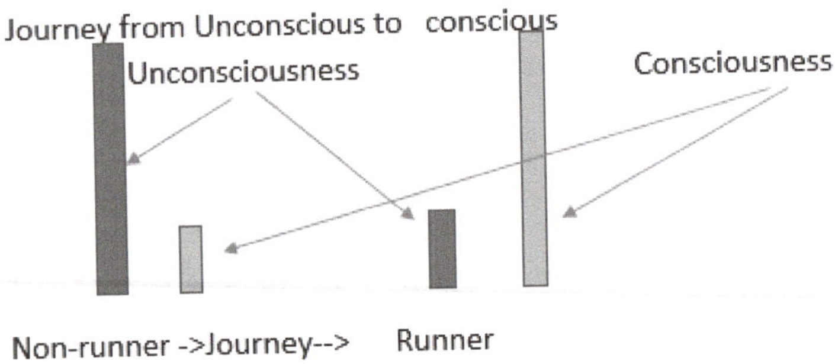

Weak decision maker--→Strong decision maker

Non-runner has bigger part of unconscious than conscious. Role of conscious in decision making process will be very small in case of non-runner though he has strong desire to begin the running in morning while going to bed. In morning at 5 am, alarm will awake you but you will find yourself unable to throw the blanket away and leave the bed because, role of conscious was very small. But in case of daily disciplined runner, role of consciousness is greater than unconsciousness therefore they throw the blanket in morning very comfortably and get ready with merry for running in out. So daily disciplined runner will be strong decision maker in other part of life too. Intoxication is the trap and has the main role for greater size of unconsciousness.

According to me, consistent running develops the hidden courage in other part of life to face any kind of new challenges with playful attitude not with seriousness. Seriousness is poison which creates tension instead of attention. Facing the any kind of challenge in life with playful attitude generates sporting feelings in which we enjoy failure and success almost equally. Tension generates the fear while attention generates awareness. Any divine effort under umbrella of awareness fetches holy fruits which is available to all to test it.

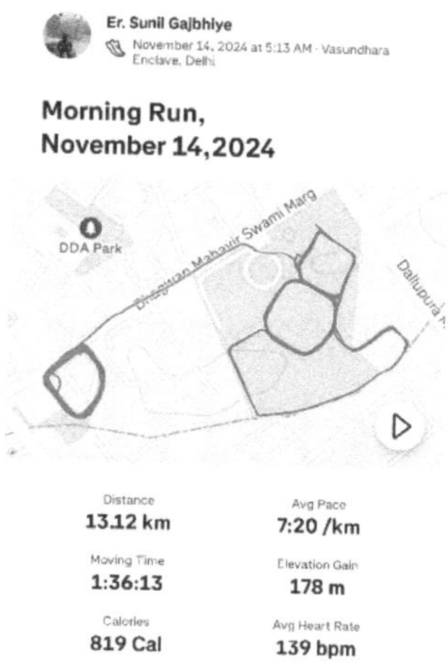
Er. Sunil Gajbhiye
November 14, 2024 at 5:13 AM · Vasundhara Enclave, Delhi
Morning Run,
November 14,2024
DDA Park
Bhagwan Mahavir Swami Marg
Distance
13.12 km
Avg Pace
7:20 /km
Moving Time
1:36:13
Elevation Gain
178 m
Calories
819 Cal
Avg Heart Rate
139 bpm

There is two type of Pain

1. Pain without cause:- Simple needle piercing in any part of body without any cause will have pain with agony.

2. Pain with cause:-Simple needle of injection by physician in any part of body to heal, will have the pain with no agony. Similarly daily running plays the role of injection to keep mind and body in healthy and peaceful condition with joyful pain.

There is old saying, "You are what you eat." But in California it's "You are what you drive, "in Italy it's "You are what you wear." and in France, "You are what you drink. But as per Runligion,"**You are what you run**" because D2 run has become the part your complacency.

(D2=Daily disciplined)

Body Boiler

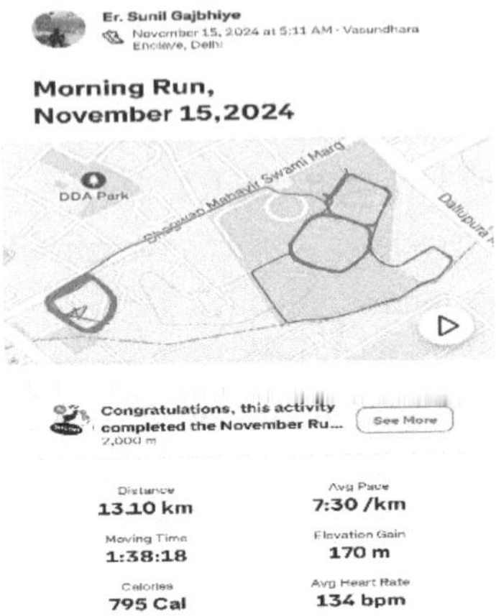
Er. Sunil Gajbhiye
November 15, 2024 at 5:11 AM · Vasundhara Enclave, Delhi
Morning Run,
November 15,2024
DDA Park
Bhagwan Mahavir Swami Marg
Congratulations, this activity completed the November Ru...
2,000 m
See More
Distance
13.10 km
Avg Pace
7:30 /km
Moving Time
1:38:18
Elevation Gain
170 m
Calories
795 Cal
Avg Heart Rate
134 bpm

Body boiler (Good Eating habit) :- In thermal power station to generate the electricity , simple process is

1. Generation of heat energy by burning the coal, food of Boiler.
2. Generation of steam by heat energy.
3. Steam generate the mechanical energy to rotate the turbo alternator to produce the electricity.

In the above process, before burning, grinding of coal is very important to increase the efficiency of boiler apart from others measures.

Same process of grinding of the food in the mouth is very important for our body as well to enhance the efficiency of our body like boiler to generate maximum useful energy. Well approximately 100% grinding of food in mouth is inevitable to reduce stress on digestive system of our body, result in night sound sleep which is very much essential for the next day blissful running with available excellent energy.

Sensible Heat (variation in temperature) and Latent Heat (Constant temperature)

During continuous heating of water we observe the temperature rising from 0 to 100 degree centigrade, this is sensible heat but temperature remains constant at 100 degree centigrade despite continuance of heating process, this heat energy called latent heat, at this stage water transform from liquid stage to gas stage i.e. steam. In the same way, Personality also has three part Solid, Liquid and gas.

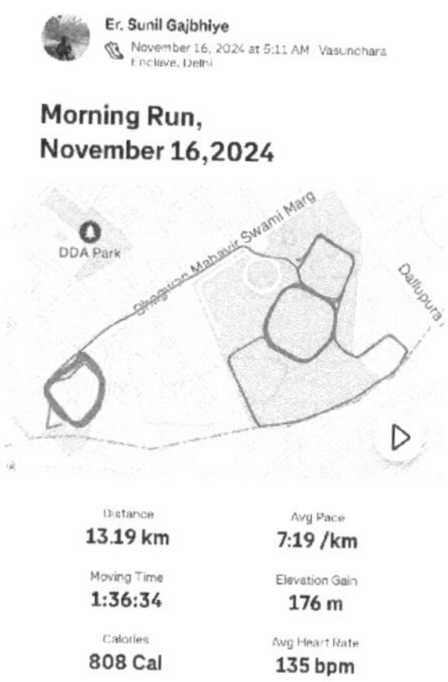
Er. Sunil Gajbhiye
November 16, 2024 at 5:11 AM · Vasundhara Enclave, Delhi
Morning Run,
November 16,2024
DDA Park
Bhagwan Mahavir Swami Marg
Dallupura
Distance
13.19 km
Avg Pace
7:19 /km
Moving Time
1:36:34
Elevation Gain
176 m
Calories
808 Cal
Avg Heart Rate
135 bpm

1. Zero running activity= Solid stage= No free movement=heaviness= No flexibility with entirely burden on society and on himself= invitation to diseases stage

2. Seldom running activity without discipline= Liquid stage= horizontal& downward free movement=flexibility with attachment= worldly stage of human with partial burden on society and himself=anxiety stage.

3. Regular Running activity with discipline=gases stage=Vertical free movement=Flexibility without attachment=supreme stage of human being and always available for philanthropy= precious blissful stage.

Solid+ Heat→ Temperature Rising (Remains in solid stage)+Heat→ Temperature constant (Transforming into liquid stage)+ Temperature rising (remains in liquid stage)+Heat→Temperature constant(Transforming into gases) . D2 running=continuous daily heating→ gradual transformation of personality.

29 km

PD=Potential difference=Voltage in electricity

Suppose you have developed the capacity to run 42 Km (marathon) twice or more in a year and you run 10 Km daily then

PD= Voltage of your body=42-10=32 km.

This voltage of 32 km running is available with you daily to utilize for any type of constructive work besides running activity.

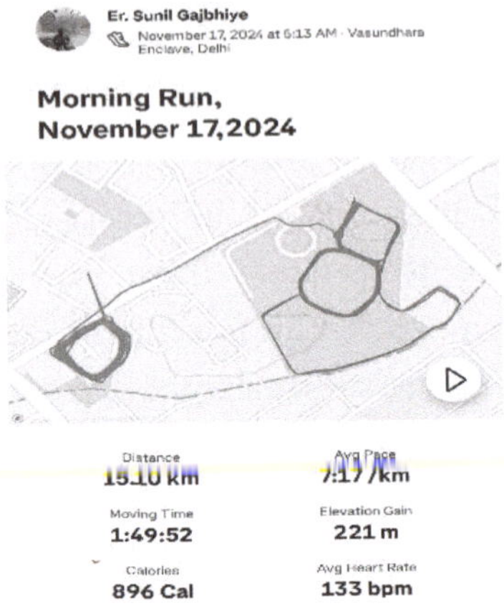

Evolvement of this notion helps to feel enjoyment during the execution of constructive work after achieving the daily running target like 10 km. Thus daily running converts the tension full effort into the tensionless effort in any execution of constructive work and then you consider the daily running as an essential tonic for your body and it becomes catalyst for next day running.

Daily disciplined running -> 3 P

1) Preparation means getting ready for running->

2) Purification means running any targeted distance ->

3) Perfection means sharing the blissfulness of post completion of targeted distance. ->

(Birth of this book is the resultant)

Monday (November 18, 2024) is rest day.

Running is the great Social work.

From *Technophelosophy* point of view social work must have two components:-

1st –Individual unit health

2nd – Society health.

Society Health= Sum of Individual health of that society.

Society health α Sum of individual health.

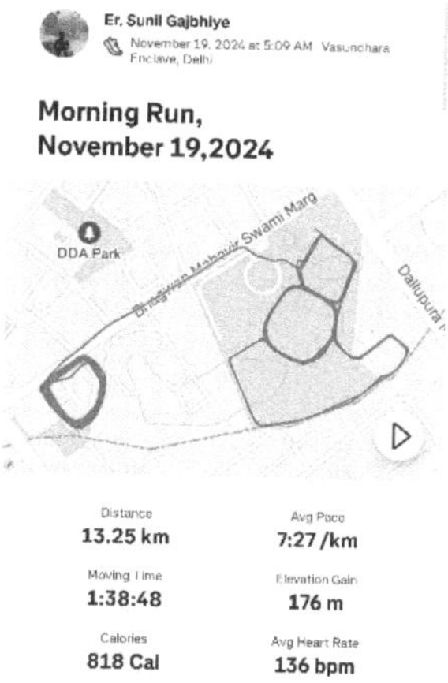

Er. Sunil Gajbhiye
November 19, 2024 at 5:09 AM Vasundhara Enclave, Delhi
Morning Run,
November 19,2024
DDA Park
Bhagwan Mahavir Swami Marg
Dallupura
Distance
13.25 km
Avg Pace
7:27 /km
Moving Time
1:38:48
Elevation Gain
176 m
Calories
818 Cal
Avg Heart Rate
136 bpm

Thus keeping oneself in good health condition must be foremost social work. Thus regular running must be great part of social work and this notion will propel you to maintain the regular discipline running as contribution toward the nation.

All organizers and individuals in world engaged in organizing the marathon events are really great and true social workers. They are directly helping the nation to become great from progress point of view.

Without 1st part of social work, imagination of social work for great nation is nothing but elusion and pretentious. Our effort to make ourselves healthy is effort to make nation healthy and for this, regular discipline running is the only great way to achieve it.

Near100% runner of society = 100 % healthy society= developed nation

50% runner of society= 50% healthy society=average developed nation.

Below 10%runner of society=10% healthy society=poor developing nation

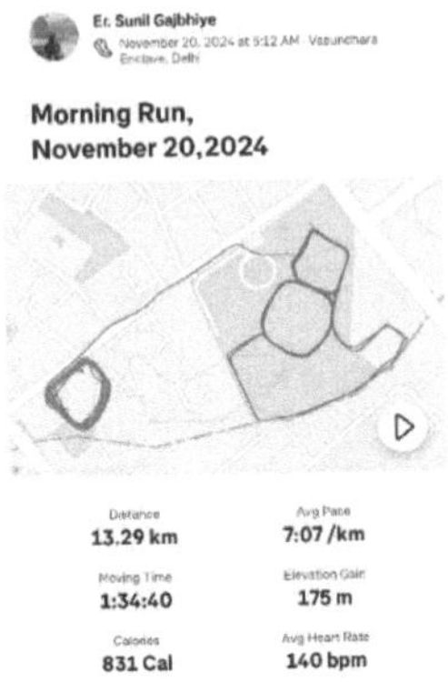
Er. Sunil Gajbhiye
November 20, 2024 at 5:12 AM · Vasundhara Enclave, Delhi
Morning Run,
November 20,2024
Distance
13.29 km
Avg Pace
7:07 /km
Moving Time
1:34:40
Elevation Gain
175 m
Calories
831 Cal
Avg Heart Rate
140 bpm

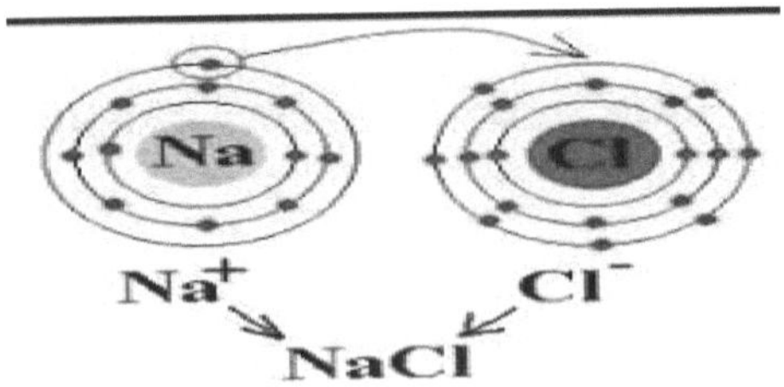

The electronic configuration of sodium chloride (NaCl) is the result of the transfer of an electron from atom of sodium to atom of chlorine, forming a sodium ion (Na+) and a chloride ion (Cl-):

- **Sodium (Na+) (positive ion)**

Sodium has an atomic number of 11 and an electronic configuration of 2, 8, 1. To achieve a full outer shell, sodium loses its one valence electron to form a sodium positive ion with an electronic configuration of 2, 8. (For overweight person losing the weight by running is achieving a full outer shell)

Technophilosophy- Loosing excess possessing material will convert the personality in positive attitude. Daily disciplined running is one of the methods of removing the negativity.

- **Chlorine (Cl-)(Negative ion)**

Chlorine has an atomic number of 17 and an electronic configuration of 2, 8, 7. To achieve a full outer shell, chlorine gains one electron to form a chlorine negative ion with an electronic configuration of 2, 8, 8. (For underweight person gaining the weight is achieving full outer shell)

Technophilosophy- Accepting and digesting others negativity enhance the immunity of the person and daily running paves path for this.

The opposite charges of the sodium and chloride ions create a strong force of attraction that binds them together to form the compound NaCl, also known as table salt.

NaCl (sodium chloride) is like utopian nation in which there is perfect balance between rich section and poor section because of which there is no place for any dissatisfaction among the public in any country. This state of perfect balance can be achieved with help of running device to pave the way towards national prosperity instead of personal prosperity.

Olympic Gold medal

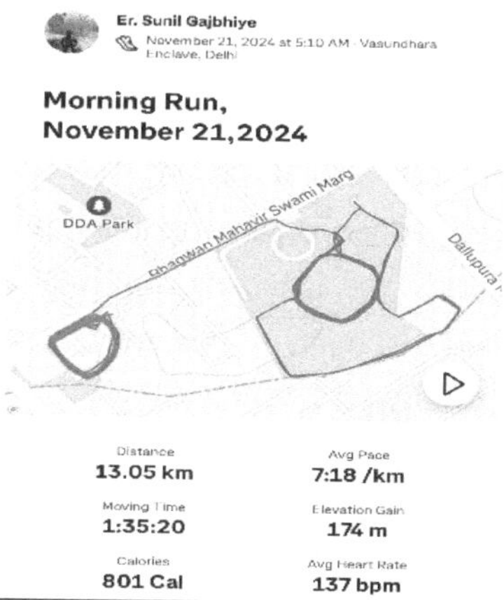
Er. Sunil Gajbhiye
November 21, 2024 at 5:10 AM · Vasundhara Enclave, Delhi
Morning Run,
November 21,2024
DDA Park
Bhagwan Mahavir Swami Marg
Distance
13.05 km
Avg Pace
7:18 /km
Moving Time
1:35:20
Elevation Gain
174 m
Calories
801 Cal
Avg Heart Rate
137 bpm

Olympic Medal Chart 2024 vs Runners'% population.

Rank	Country	Gold	Silver	Bronze	Total	Runners'%
1	US	40	44	42	126	15%
2	China	40	27	24	91	21%
3	Japan	20	12	13	45	8.6%
4	Australia	18	19	16	53	11%
5	France	16	26	22	64	25%
71	India	0	1	5	6	0.14%

My interpretation from above data is, all top five countries are having apt great number of runners, have made the place in top five. In this regard India's position is thinkable as per chart. It implies that involvement of maximum people in running activity will create the fertile soil for the athletes to fetch the maximum medals for the country. Creating the atmosphere of running in the country is like preparation by ploughing the crop field for the future medals. For this, making the running activity compulsory subject right from the 1st standards of all schools in the country is inevitable for making place in top five in future. This is like SIP investment which will have great significant return after 20 years. Running is the least expensive and convenience activity so anybody can afford it irrespective of his economic status.

33 km

Maruti 800

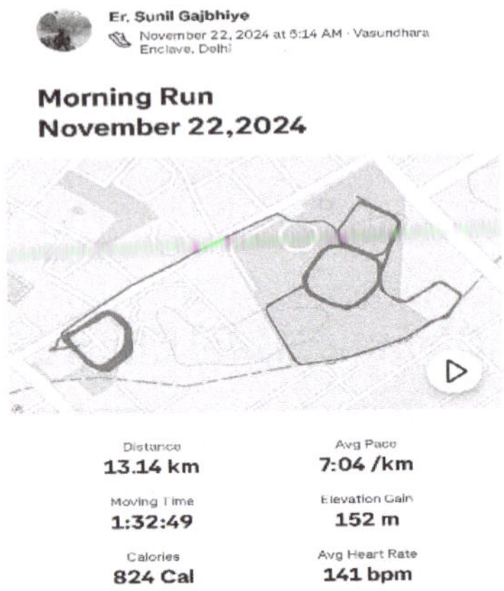
Er. Sunil Gajbhiye
November 22, 2024 at 5:14 AM · Vasundhara Enclave, Delhi
Morning Run
November 22,2024
Distance
13.14 km
Avg Pace
7:04 /km
Moving Time
1:32:49
Elevation Gain
152 m
Calories
824 Cal
Avg Heart Rate
141 bpm

We cannot tow the truck by Maruti 800 because engine capacity of maruti 800 will not be capable to pull the truck of heavy load mechanically. Regular excess load on engine of Maruti 800 beyond its capacity will reduce the life of it .This is applicable to our body as well. Our heart is like engine of Maruti 800 and our overweight will be like towing the truck of heavy load to Maruti 800 which will caused unnecessary overload on the heart which is against system of nature. Regular running regulates the body weight and helps to maintain it near good BMI.

Maintaining the good BMI is possible by daily disciplined running with parallel good healthy diet system and thus mostly we can keep ourselves away from heart related problems. To achieve the good BMI we need to become the disciple of D2 running which helps to become spiritually powerful because each disciplined run teaches us something unique lesson if it is with awareness. Disciplined run with awareness is a unique part of meditation.

Type of fear

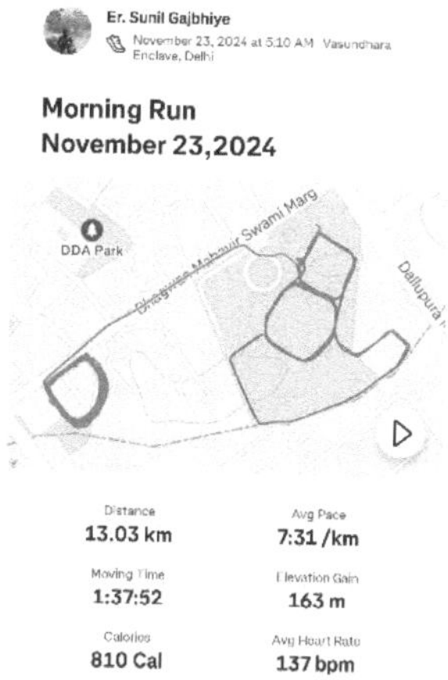
Er. Sunil Gajbhiye
November 23, 2024 at 5:10 AM Vasundhara Enclave, Delhi
Morning Run
November 23,2024
DDA Park
Swami Marg
Distance
13.03 km
Avg Pace
7:31 /km
Moving Time
1:37:52
Elevation Gain
163 m
Calories
810 Cal
Avg Heart Rate
137 bpm

- **Natural Fear:** - This fear is for the survival and is common trait in all animals. This fear makes all animals to protect themselves from any kind of calamity in their life. This fear is the great gift of nature to all animals. Knowing this fear is the first step toward awareness. The presence of this fear develops idea in mind to be aware of all odds happening around us.
- **Artificial Fear:** - This fear is the part of only human being. Human being first amasses the money and material more than his requirement and after that fear of losing even the small part of the excess money and material is come in existence. This is the artificial fear. Because of this fear human being enters the vicious circle and excess artificial fear is the mother of superstition, result in absence of the peace which is real ornament of human being.
- **Without peace of mind, all possessing wealth = zero value**

Natural fear may develop the great willingness towards the daily running, why? Fear of getting sick may compel one to adopt the natural exercise running. So let the natural fear enter in our daily life and let it work as catalyst for D2 running and keep us away from artificial fear which is the part of vicious circle. D2 Running is like the regulator between naturals fear and artificial fear. It is also like "Journey from artificial fear to natural fear."

Natural Fear:-

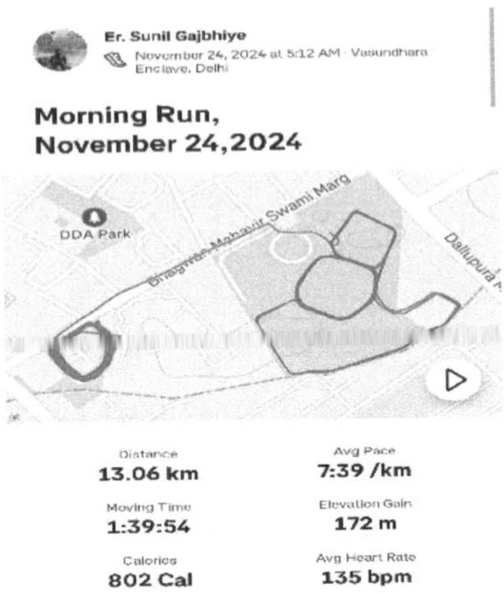
Er. Sunil Gajbhiye
November 24, 2024 at 5:12 AM · Vasundhara Enclave, Delhi
Morning Run,
November 24,2024
DDA Park
Bhagwan Mahavir Swami Marg
Distance
13.06 km
Avg Pace
7:39 /km
Moving Time
1:39:54
Elevation Gain
172 m
Calories
802 Cal
Avg Heart Rate
135 bpm

Hens and birds both have the wings but we will not see any hen or cock flying in the sky why?

According to technophilosophy, almost all flying birds' lay their eggs in nest built on the branch of trees. Hatching process by birds completed on the branches of tree at some level above the ground. After some fixed days, baby birds born in the nest and mother birds arranged their food for few days. After few fixed days, the wings of bird developed enough to fly, but in initial stage during the first falling of baby bird from nest, generates the natural fear feeling to survive and it starts to use the developed wing to fly and succeeds after few attempts. Contrary hen lay their eggs on the ground and chick doesn't get that opportunity to generate the natural fear feeling of falling, result in no flying in the sky despite having wings. Since there is no flying activity of hen, its body weight become enough heavier than the capacity of its wings to fly in sky which develops the great resistance to attempt to fly in sky.

There must be natural fear feeling for good health to generate the intangible wings for flying in world of D2 running.

Monday (November 25, 2024) is rest day.

36 km

Daily running activity is like SIP or RD for future healthy state of body. It start paying back dividend from the age of 90 years in form of reduction of bedridden period of old age.

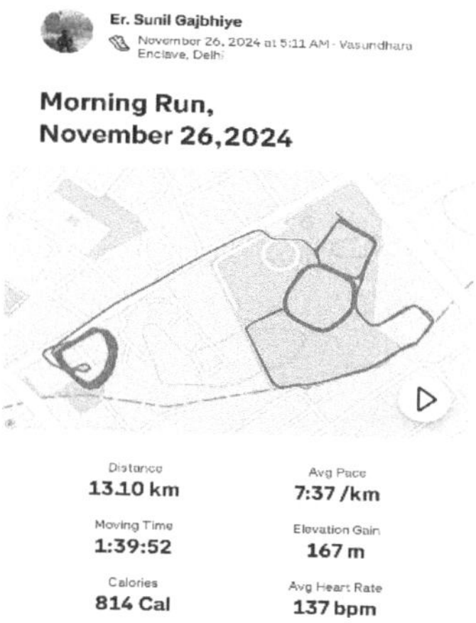

Er. Sunil Gajbhiye
November 26, 2024 at 5:11 AM · Vasundhara Enclave, Delhi
Morning Run, November 26,2024
Distance
13.10 km
Avg Pace
7:37 /km
Moving Time
1:39:52
Elevation Gain
167 m
Calories
814 Cal
Avg Heart Rate
137 bpm

RD= Running daily =Recurring deposit.

Unique and inexpressible feeling during daily running perishes feeling of being old, which provides you to be active in personal or public life because healthy body is the abode of the healthy mind.

Daily running ->feeling of youngness

Idleness means no running, causes rusting in the body which leads to n number of unknown and known diseases which are curable and incurable as well. No daily running habit beget the feeling of being old specifically after 60 years.

No running->feeling of oldness

D2 running→feeling of youngness aura

So today's investment in form of daily running is the future dividend in form of health body means least burden on himself, family, society and nation.

Technophilosophical Classification of workforce in any organization.

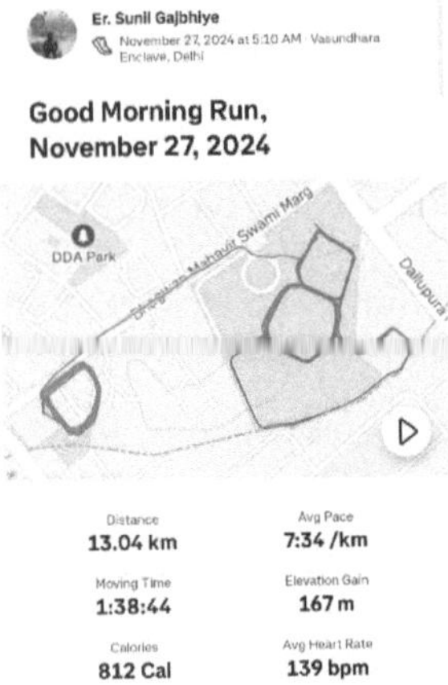
Er. Sunil Gajbhiye
November 27, 2024 at 5:10 AM · Vasundhara Enclave, Delhi
Good Morning Run, November 27, 2024
DDA Park
Bhagwan Mahavir Swami Marg
Dallupura
Distance
13.04 km
Avg Pace
7:34 /km
Moving Time
1:38:44
Elevation Gain
167 m
Calories
812 Cal
Avg Heart Rate
139 bpm

- *Energy* = Input (2+3) = 5(Output), Equation for combination of 2 group of runners and non-runners.
- *Synergy*= Input (2+3) =6 (output), Equation for group of all runners,
- *Denergy*=Input(2+3)= 4 (output), Equation for group of all non-runners

First Equation for *Energy (E1)* - Assuming in any organization for given task, combination of employee having two group (a) Runners and (b) non-runner with equal skill then as per first equation result will be near **Input=output** because high efficiency of runners will compensate low efficiency of nonrunners. Skill always needs the help of efficiency to get desired result.

Second Equation for *Synergy (E2)*- Assuming in any organization for given task, all employees are runner then as per second equation result will be near **Input<output** because high efficiency of whole workforce of runners will be in one direction of high voltage and here (E2) will be greater than (E1) and hence will have better result than (E1).

Third equation for *Denergy (E3)*- Assuming in any organization for given task, all employees are nonrunner then as per third equation result will be near **Input>output** because of absence of runner's efficiency in working force and here (E3) will be least output provider, despite skill workforce.

(E3)<(E1)<(E2) =Low tension(Voltage)< medium tension(Voltage)<High tension(Voltage) (refer to voltage section of 30 km)

Therefore all organization must be emphasized on daily running activity of their employee right from top to bottom for good quality and quantity of result, of course it will be very tough task in the beginning of implementation but over the period it will become the beautiful device of organization. This device will be very useful to perish the servility in the organization which is the most dangerous obstacle for the fast and smooth progression.

In electrical Engineering, $P = I^2 * R$

P= Power Dissipated in circuit

I = Current

R= Resistance

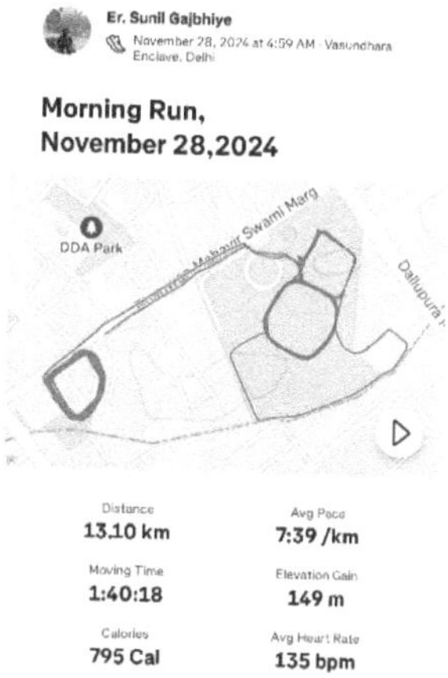
Er. Sunil Gajbhiye
November 28, 2024 at 4:59 AM · Vasundhara Enclave, Delhi
Morning Run,
November 28,2024
DDA Park
Swami Marg
Distance
13.10 km
Avg Pace
7:39 /km
Moving Time
1:40:18
Elevation Gain
149 m
Calories
795 Cal
Avg Heart Rate
135 bpm

This dissipated power in filament of bulb transformed into heat energy and then radiates light.

In running world, daily running is the analog of current I, R is the natural resistance of mind because of tendency of lying in comfort zone and overcoming the resistance result in consistent blissful journey toward the enlightenment. Therefore D_2 running is device/touchstone against any aberration in mind and defies the status quo due to fear.

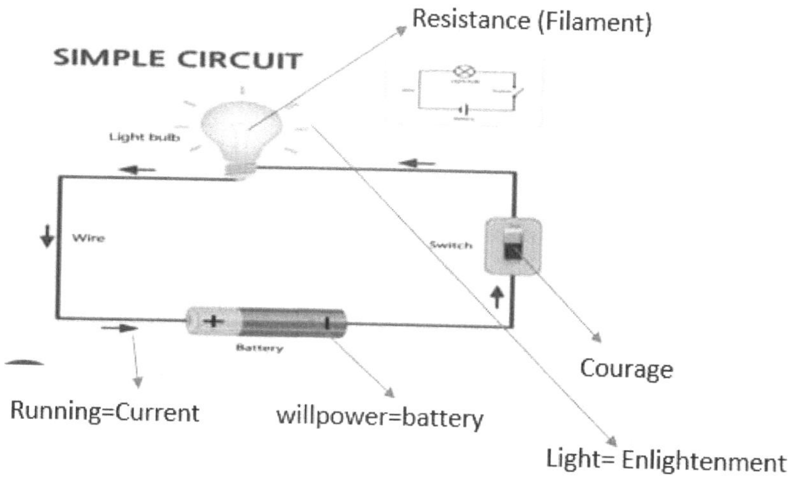

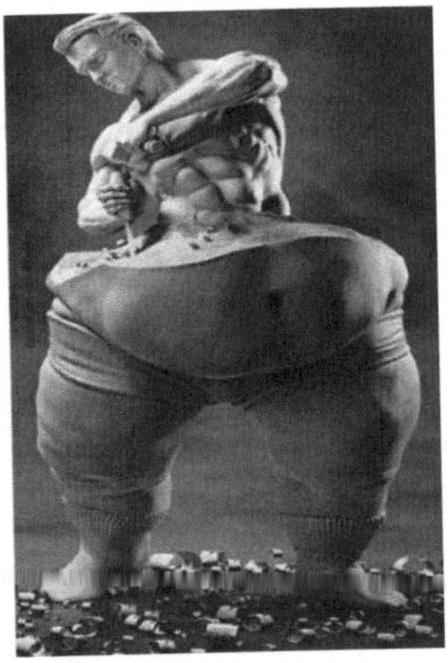

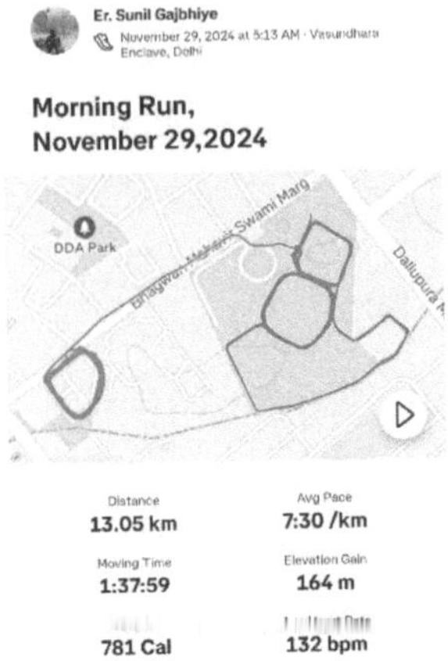

Be the self- carving Sculptor of your own body.

What is sculpting?

Removing the unnecessary outer portion by chipping from any stone to give the shape of statue of imagination. Similarly we must shape our body as per natural size by adopting daily running activity in our life. D2 running activity is removing the unnecessary portion from our body. During breathing and eating we intake combination of necessary and unnecessary element. Necessary and useful elements are for being in state of good health while unnecessary dangerous and futile elements are to destroy the state of good natural health. D2 running is to give the direction to essential elements to use them for the betterment of body while at the same time daily running helps to consume or burn the dangerous harmful elements in the body because of contaminated intake . Thus D2 running is the almost panacea for our body and also helps to attune with existence.

Daily disciplined running → Utilization of essential elements
→ Burning of dangerous harmful elements

40 km

According to Technophilosophy

Brain = Hardware= Noun

Mind = Software=Verb

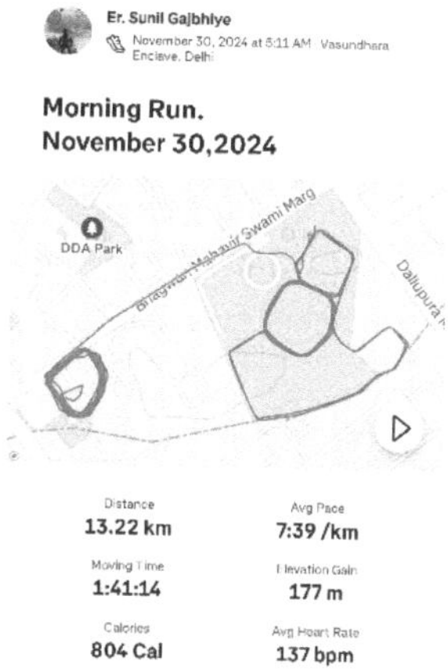
Er. Sunil Gajbhiye
November 30, 2024 at 5:11 AM Vasundhara Enclave, Delhi
Morning Run.
November 30,2024
DDA Park
Swami Marg
Dallupura
Distance
13.22 km
Avg Pace
7:39 /km
Moving Time
1:41:14
Elevation Gain
177 m
Calories
804 Cal
Avg Heart Rate
137 bpm

Regular maintenance of hardware is inevitable because it is like rail track on which train run smoothly and in case of poor maintenance of rail track, possibility of derailed of the train in future cannot be rule out. Mind as software is use for programing which give the direction to other limbs of body to execute the work generated in brain. Healthy software will always keen to absorb good programing while unhealthy software would eager to absorb unwanted programing. Unwanted programing is the good relative of procrastination while good programing is the good relative of watchfulness.

D2 running is the daily preventive maintenance of all limbs of our body including brain (most important hardware) to keep them in healthy condition which pave the path for generation of good programing of software. This is all the real treasure that we have been endowed with. D2 running prevents you from parasite state.

Good programing means installation of helping attitude which is first milestone for the country to become Nation and D2 running among the citizens may be proved beautiful instrument in this context.

“Being ignorant is not so much shame, as being unwilling to learn”

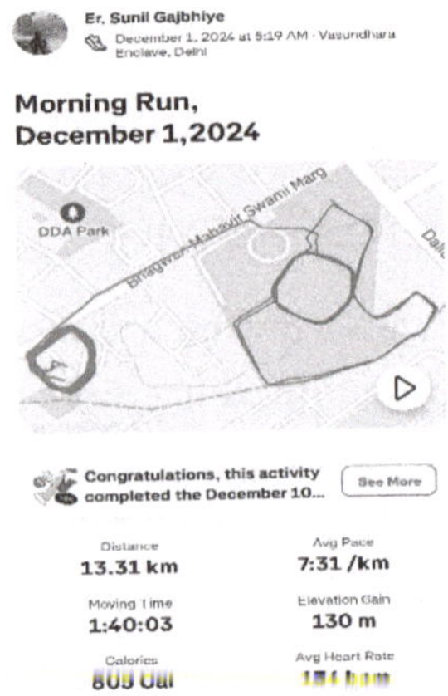
Er. Sunil Gajbhiye
December 1, 2024 at 5:19 AM · Vasundhara Enclave, Delhi
Morning Run,
December 1,2024
DDA Park
Bhagwan Mahavir Swami Marg
Congratulations, this activity completed the December 10...
See More
Distance
13.31 km
Avg Pace
7:31 /km
Moving Time
1:40:03
Elevation Gain
130 m
Calories
Avg Heart Rate

There are many types of therapy, including psychotherapy, counseling, speech therapy, physical therapy, and more. According to today's thought during running, D2 Running is the only one kind of the physical therapy which has further two types:

1) Post Therapy: Treatment after occurrence of disease.

2) Pre therapy: Treatment before occurrence of disease.

Post therapy like running or walking after the advice of physician is the common scenario in parks or sport complex. More than 90% walkers come under this type of therapy. The walkers or runners under this category, are generally indiscipline and irregular in their activity.

Pre therapy is daily running without advice of physician and their population is less than 10% in various parks and sport complexes.

The walkers or runners under this category, are generally disciplined and very regular in their activity. When Pre physical therapy becomes the part of daily amusement then it is achievement of state of the sainthood. Daily running as part of pre therapy is to hone the skill of concentration, to enhance remembrance power, sane and decisiveness which are very helpful in day to day constructive work.

Running period = Hermit period

Running place= Hermitage

"Prevention is better than cure"

Motivational Zone

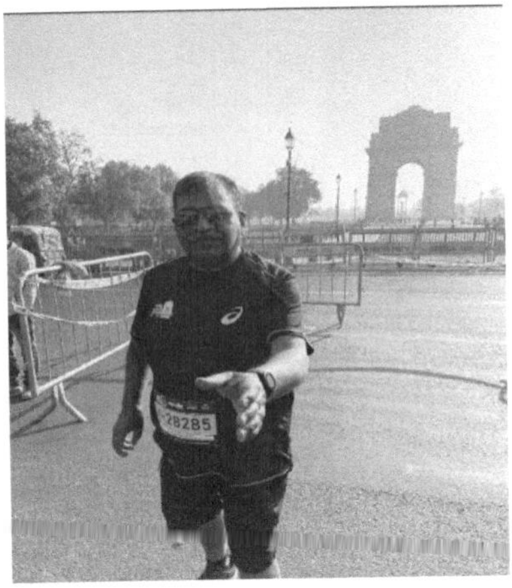

A retired senior bank officer, an active voice in the matters of his community, a devoted husband and father of three well-established children, Mr. Bhim Singh Kapil never got much time to indulge in any sort of fitness throughout his life. However, after the retirement from his services, and seeking new hobbies, he began coming to Chilla Sports Complex in Vasundhara Enclave on a regular basis. This was a time when our friendship developed, and, **I encouraged and successfully motivated to Mr. Kapil to start running from the age of 62 with weight of around 90** kg. In November 2023, At the age of 65 just a few months after our first meetings, he participated in his first 10k Run in Rishikesh (Uttrakhand) in hilly area with great elevation. Who would imagine his perseverance would take him to complete multiple running events within a year, including half-marathons(**21** km) such as SMVD Katra Marathon in Katra, Jammu (April 2024), Vedanta Half Marathon in Delhi (October 2024), Tata Mumbai Half Marathon (January 2025), and the Apollo Tyre Delhi Half Marathon (February 2025).

It was far from an easy journey - although young at heart, Mr. Kapil had to overcome the challenges expected for his age, control his diabetes and weight, to gather the physical and mental endurance required to face long running distances under the often unforgiving hot weather of North India, or the extreme humidity of Mumbai.

Mr Kapil's resilience and vigor have been remarkable - even after many years of a hectic and fulfilling career and family life, he has overcome his own physical limitations and rudimentary knowledge of fitness to embrace a new and exciting journey towards a healthier, more active lifestyle. His willingness to embrace a new chapter of self-improvement and discipline at a senior stage of his life is a remarkable example that shall inspire every Indian, regardless of age and rudimentary body weight physical fitness or lifestyle.

Finish Line touching of real life Marathon

"From hospital bed to starting line — a journey of heart and hope."
Running, fitness, and an active life were part of my DNA. As a practicing General Physician and a fitness lover, I thrived on aerobics, gym workouts, swimming laps, smashing shuttlecocks on the badminton court, and feeling the ground rush under my feet during a run. But three years ago, an unexpected diagnosis — cancer of the floor of the mouth — forced me off the track. A major surgery involving jaw resection and reconstruction left me unable to even walk steadily. The fighter in me realized: this was not the finish line, but the starting point of a new race.

The early steps were painful and slow, like the grueling first miles of a marathon against a fierce headwind. Yet every small achievement — standing, walking, moving without help — became a personal finish line worth celebrating. I built my strength from the ground up, just like a runner prepares for a race: patiently, persistently, with heart. Walking turned into jogging, jogging into running, and running into reclaiming my life. Gym sessions returned, badminton racquets came alive, swimming lanes reopened — and with each comeback, I gained more than just fitness; I gained unshakable faith.

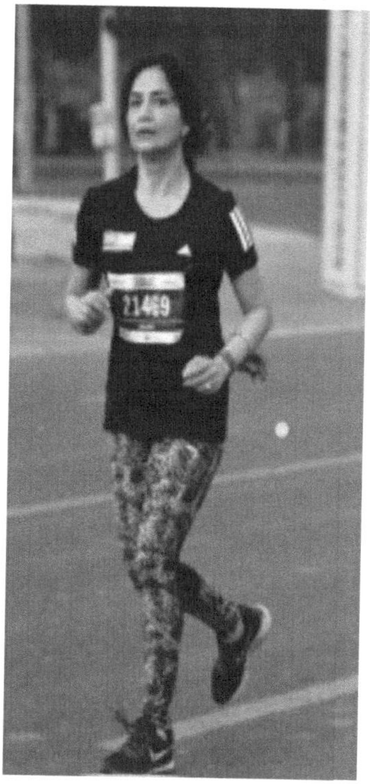

Today, I lace up my shoes not just to run, but to honor the journey. Cancer tried to sideline me, but it only deepened my love for movement, life, and resilience. The race never ends — we just find new ways to run it, stronger each time.

– Dr Abhilasha Agarwal

Ms. Sandhya: Age 60

A Journey of Grit, Grace & Glory

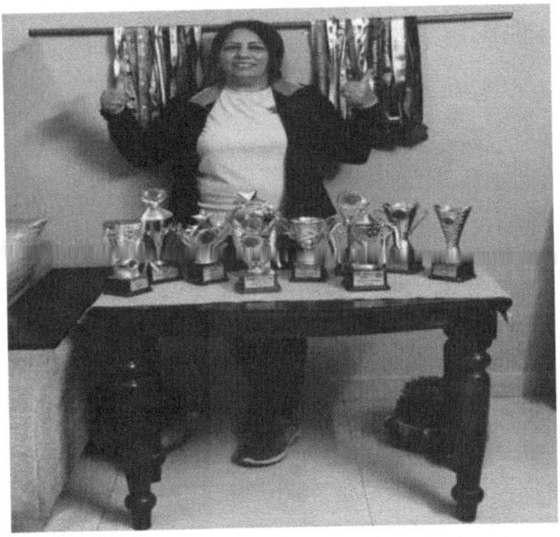

Ms. Sandhya is a spirited mother of two accomplished daughters, known for her infectious laughter, boundless generosity, and a heart that beats for those around her. Beneath her graceful demeanor lies a playful, loving inner child—ever eager to nurture, ever ready to give. Life, however, hasn't always been kind. In 2009 what began as a seemingly harmless stomach ache unraveled into a life-altering diagnosis: stage 4 stomach lymphoma. With five rounds of chemotherapy and a major surgery as her only shot at survival, Ms. Sandhya was thrust into a battle she never saw coming. Pain, fear, and uncertainty ruled her days—but she never let them win.

Against all odds, she made it through. And when she did, she made a promise to herself: that every single breath would count. What started as gentle walks post-recovery evolved into full-blown marathon training. Today, Ms. Sandhya is not just a survivor—she's a decorated marathoner with over 250medals,trophies and certificates, a living testament to discipline, resilience, and the sheer will to rise. She's conquered marathons in some of the most breathtaking yet challenging terrains—Mashobra, Katra, Rishikesh, Mumbai, Ladakh, and more.

Her journey has earned her the Runner of the Year award just last year, and first prize in multiple prestigious Runs, along with recognition through significant cash prizes. But Ms. Sandhya doesn't just run—she lives with full vibrancy. She dances through Zumba and aerobics, treks across mountains, stirs magic in the kitchen, and sings with a voice that's as joyful as her spirit. She is the definition of multi-dimensional strength and unstoppable energy.

Ms. Sandhya's story is not just one of survival—it is one of complete rebirth. Her life is a masterclass in turning pain into purpose. She proves that even after life knocks you down, you can rise stronger, laugh louder, and run farther. She is the embodiment of what it means to not just heal, but to thrive—reminding us all that with hope in your heart and purpose in your stride, anything is possible.

Yes, I Can": My Journey from Bedridden to Marathon Runner

By Vidushi Karnatak

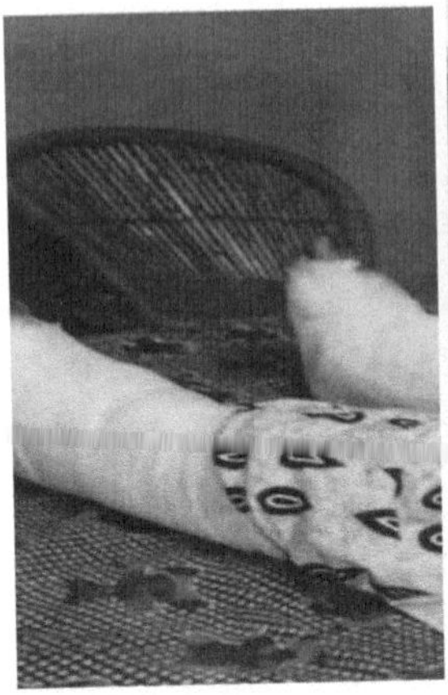

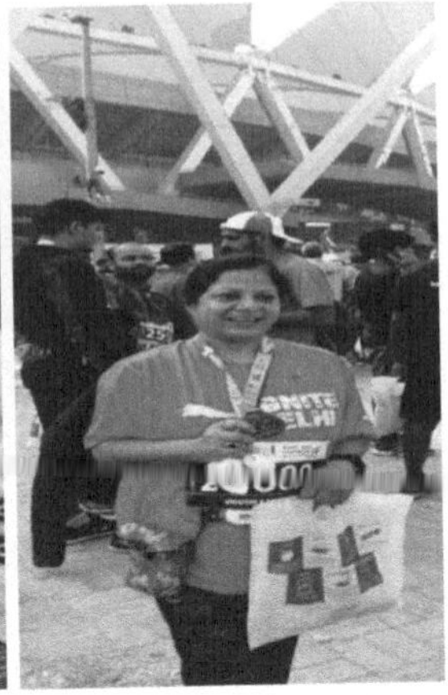

Life has a way of testing our limits, often in the most unexpected ways. A few years ago, I found myself facing one of the biggest challenges of my life—a major accident that left me completely bedridden. The damage was severe. Screws had to be inserted in both my legs, and the simple act of walking became a distant dream.

For 3 to 4 months, I couldn't even stand. The pain was physical, but the real battle was mental—fighting fear, helplessness, and the temptation to give up. But deep within, I made a choice. I told myself, "Vidushi, you're not done yet."

Instead of surrendering to despair, I embraced a new mantra: Yes, I Can.

My journey to recovery began slowly, with baby steps, quite literally. The road was long and often lonely, but I had a vision—to walk again, to run again, and to reclaim not just my mobility, but my life.

Chilla Sports Complex became my sanctuary. With each visit, I challenged my limits—first with slow walks, then brisk ones, and eventually, something I never imagined: running. Today, I proudly participate in both half and full marathons.

The inspiration for running was given By Sh. Devender Aroraji and Sh.Sunil Gajbhiyeji, who were prolific runners and even running today. They even inspired my husband Sh. Ashutosh Karnatak, to run and with me he also participates in the marathons.

People often ask me what kept me going. The answer is simple: Positivity, Purpose, and Perseverance. I refused to let an accident define my future. Every setback carries the seed of a comeback—if only we choose to nurture it.

To anyone facing adversity—whether physical, emotional, or mental—I say this: You are stronger than you think. Don't let circumstances dictate your spirit. Embrace your pain, honour your struggle, and rise with resilience.

If I can run marathons with screws in both my legs, then truly, nothing is impossible.

Remember, "Yes, You Can" – Challenge your Limitations – Try it… be a runner too.

My Running Journey – Poonam Agarwal

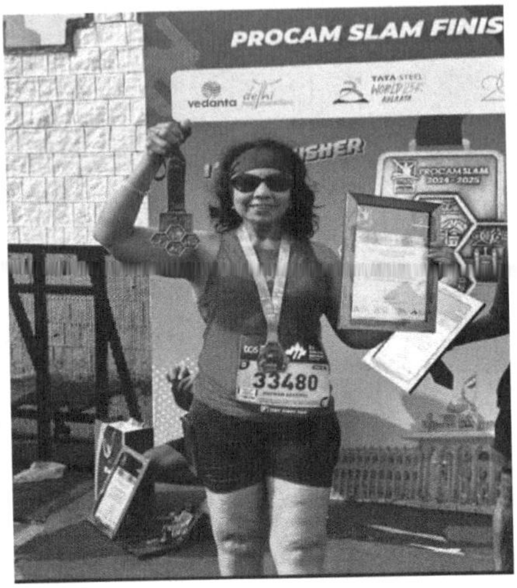

I'm Poonam Agarwal, and my journey as a runner began at a time when I was struggling with weight and several health issues. Determined to take charge of my health, I started with simple brisk walks. One day, my daughters encouraged me to participate in the Pinkathon and run just 3 kilometers. I agreed—and crossing that first finish line became a pivotal moment in my life. From that day forward, there was no turning back. It has now been nearly a decade since I first laced up my running shoes.

Today, I am a proud member of RunXpress, a vibrant running group, where I also serve as a captain. I've had the honor of leading at events like Soldierathon and representing multiple prestigious marathons as an ambassador—these include the SMVD Katra Marathon, Piku Sports, the Ganga Sustainability Run, Runex Sports, and many others.

Over the years, I have participated in more than 200 events and have been fortunate to win over 50 podium trophies, in addition to numerous awards as a RunXpress captain and ambassador.

Recently, I was deeply honored to be felicitated by Lt. Gen. Shankar Narayan PVSM, NM, VSM, Commandant of ARHH, New Delhi. Another significant milestone was completing the Procam Slam, which includes four major races across India:

Vedanta Delhi Half Marathon – 21 km

Tata Steel Kolkata 25K – 25 km

Tata Mumbai Marathon – 42 km

TCS World 10K Bengaluru – 10 km

My Procam journey was filled with emotional and physical challenges. On the day of the Delhi Half Marathon, it coincided with Karva Chauth. Observing the traditional fast, I ran 21 kilometers without food or water. It tested not just my endurance but my spirit.

Later, after completing the grueling 42 km Mumbai Marathon, life took a devastating turn. My husband was admitted to the ICU, where he fought for his life for a month. He passed away on February 26. Amidst overwhelming grief and exhaustion, I still had one final race left in my Procam journey. Though my heart was heavy and my body weak, I pushed forward. I ran not just for myself, but in honor of my husband's memory and the dreams we once shared.

Completing the Procam Slam wasn't just about running races—it was about resilience, love, and the unshakable will to keep going, even when everything seems to fall apart.

There are many girls such as Poonam Verma,Sunita ,Rekha ,Neha ,Ruma,Jyoti, Pinky,Mahua,Richa, who are inspired by me & joined with me

Journey from pain to pen by Mr. Ramender Guleria

"Stroke. Crash. Comeback. — I Wasn't Built to Break."

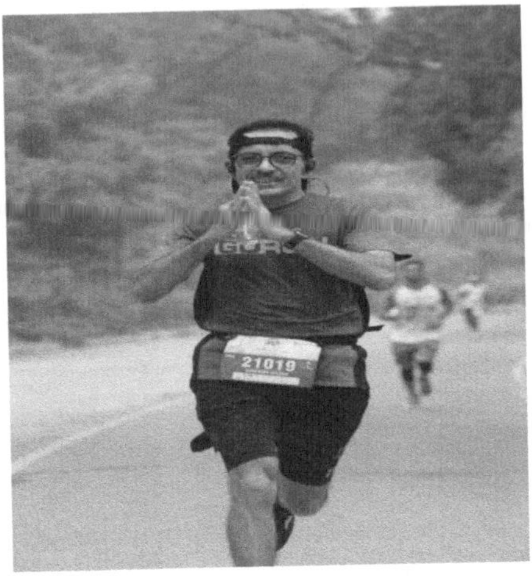

In 2005, I was climbing the corporate ladder — grinding, hustling, chasing targets. Then a stroke hit me like a lightning bolt. Just 30, and I was paralyzed on my left side. Recovery took two months, but the damage was deeper — I lost my job, my routine, my rhythm.

Eventually, I got back on my feet... and straight back into the rat race. No time for health. Just deadlines and deliverables. Until life hit pause again. Stroke #2. In 2015. This time, recovery was faster — 25 days. But the doctors didn't mince words:

"Change your lifestyle, or you won't survive the next one."

That was the turning point.

I started cycling when I could squeeze in time. Then in 2016, I took the boldest decision of my life — I left my job and started my own business. With freedom came clarity. And with clarity came running.

From struggling to complete 5Ks to training with seasoned runners — I found a new rhythm. My weekends became about bibs and medals, not meetings and boardrooms. I ran everything:

Airtel/Vedanta Half Marathons, New Delhi Marathon, Super Sikh, Aravali Hills, Coach Ravinder's races, even the brutal Ladakh Marathon in 2017 and again in 2023.

But then — plot twist.

In June 2023, my knees gave out. I ran Ladakh HM and Vedanta in excruciating pain. Finally, I surrendered. Knee surgery in Dec 2023. Bed rest. Physiotherapy. And a terrifying thought: Will I ever run again?

I almost quit.

But then… I remembered who I am.

I started slow. Walking. Jogging. Researched recovery like my life depended on it. Strength training. Rehab. Discipline. Support from fellow runners.

In Feb 2024, I ran my first post-surgery Half Marathon.

In April, I conquered a 10K hill run in Katra.

And since then — I've won 19 trophies across 5K, 10K, 16K, and 21K races.

But this comeback mindset didn't begin in 2016.

Back in college, I was a thrill-seeker — I did 3 years of horse riding, tent pegging, and show jumping in Udhampur and Dharamshala. Then joined the Naval Hang Gliding Club — flying over cliffs, chasing wind currents. I competed in the Inter-Defence Hang Gliding Championship in Vizag and ranked 7th.

Until another life-altering moment:

A major crash during a gliding expedition off Tirupati hills.

Rescued by a Naval helicopter.

Two broken ribs. Pierced my heart. Doctors gave me 24 hours. Then another 24.

I survived those too.

So here I am. Not because I never fell — but because I never stayed down.

To everyone out there battling injuries, burnout, or self-doubt — know this:

You're not broken. You're rebuilding.

Your scars aren't your weakness — they're proof that you healed.

And your best chapter? It's not behind you — it's the comeback you're writing right now.

Guleria

Chapter Title: A Decade on the Run

Prashant Tandon

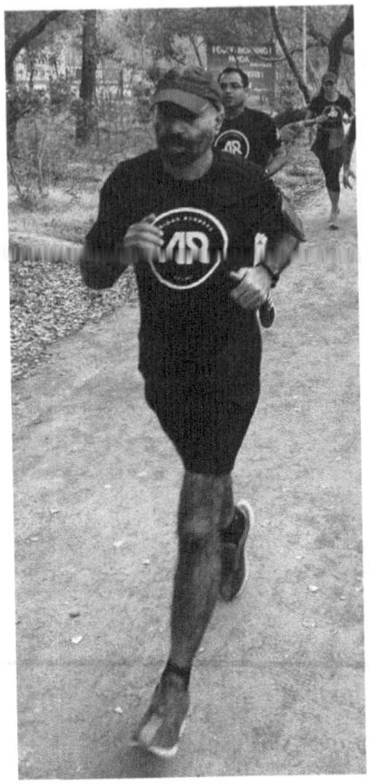

In 2025, I celebrate ten years since I began running marathons. A full decade. I'm now 60, but remarkably, my energy hasn't waned the way most people expect it to at this age. I believe that's largely because I run. Running marathons demands consistency, discipline, and resilience—qualities that have not only shaped my fitness but also my way of life.

Preparing for a marathon is no part-time commitment. It requires training every day, year-round. This kind of dedication forces structure into your routine—early mornings at the track, mindful eating, regular stretching, and cross-training through cycling or swimming. The payoff? Not just a healthy body, but a disciplined life.

An Accidental Beginning

I didn't grow up with a passion for long-distance running. In fact, my athletic journey began with hockey during my student days. But when I entered the world of journalism in the late 1980s, physical activity gradually faded from my life. The job demanded long, irregular hours and left little room for a consistent fitness routine. Occasionally, I made time for the gym, but nothing more.

Then, in 2015, everything changed.

Two close friends, Devender Arora and Sunil Gajbhiye (who is also the author of this book), nudged me toward something unexpected. They were regulars at the Chilla Sports Complex and encouraged me to sign up for an upcoming 10-kilometre race. I registered somewhat hesitantly, unsure of what I was getting into.

That first race was both humbling and exhilarating. I crossed the finish line in 1 hour and 15 minutes. Tired but proud, I felt something stir within me. A challenge had been thrown, and I was ready to take it on.

RunXpress and the Road Ahead

That 10K run gave me the confidence to aim higher. Later that season, I registered for a half marathon. Around this time, I met Devendra Arora ji—fondly known as "Captain" in the running community. He became my mentor and introduced me to a new way of training.

Under his guidance, I joined his running group, *RunXpress*. It was through this group that I learned about tempo runs, interval training, and proper running technique. Together, we explored almost every running track in Delhi. The camaraderie, the shared goals, the sense of belonging—it all deepened my commitment to the sport.

My First Half Marathon

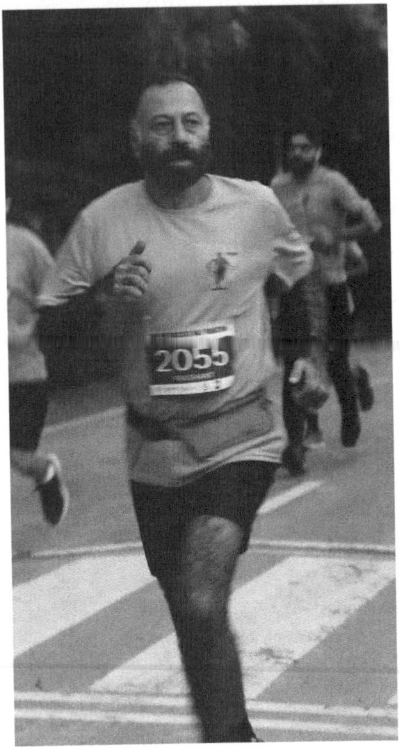

The Airtel Delhi Half Marathon, 2015 was my first official 21-kilometre race. I completed it with a beginner's timing of 2 hours and 30 minutes. But that number didn't matter as much as what it represented: perseverance, growth, and the beginning of a new identity.

I was no longer just a journalist. I was a runner.

Setback and Comeback

In December 2023, life tested me in an entirely new way.

While returning from the stadium one evening, I met with a serious accident. I suffered a skull fracture, a torn rotator cuff, and six broken ribs. The pain was excruciating, but worse than the physical injuries was the sudden halt to my momentum.

For five months, I was confined to bed. Every small movement was a challenge. But even during those dark days, my mind kept returning to the track. The mental strength that marathon running had instilled in me became my lifeline.

By July and August of 2024, I started walking in the park. Slowly, painfully, I worked my way up to running 2–3 kilometers. Each step felt like a victory. By the end of the year, I was back where I belonged—running. I even completed two half marathons after my recovery.

The accident could have ended my running story. Instead, it added a new chapter—one of resilience, healing, and the power of a never-give-up mindset.

Running as a Way of Life

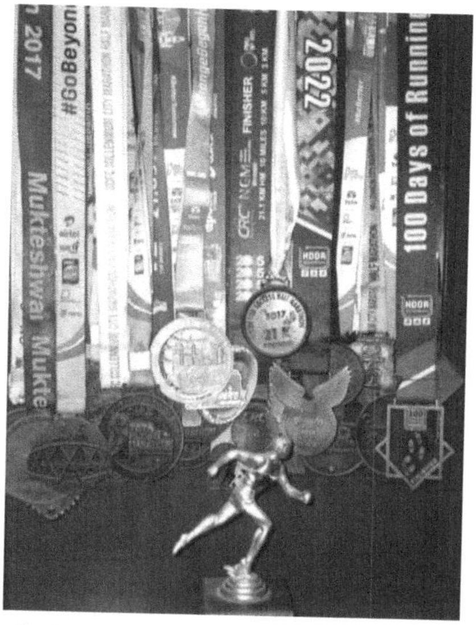

Marathon running has taught me lessons that extend far beyond the road. The most important of them: I am only competing with myself. I don't get discouraged when others run ahead. I focus on my own pace, my own progress. My goal is simple—to be better than I was yesterday.

Running has also gifted me something beautiful: a chance to witness the soul of different cities during their quietest, most serene hours. Whether in India or abroad, the early morning streets—empty, glowing with the first light of day—feel like a private world reserved just for runners.

And all it takes is a pair of running shoes, some shorts, and a T-shirt.

Passengers of Tranquility Train at Chilla Sport Complex Delhi, India.

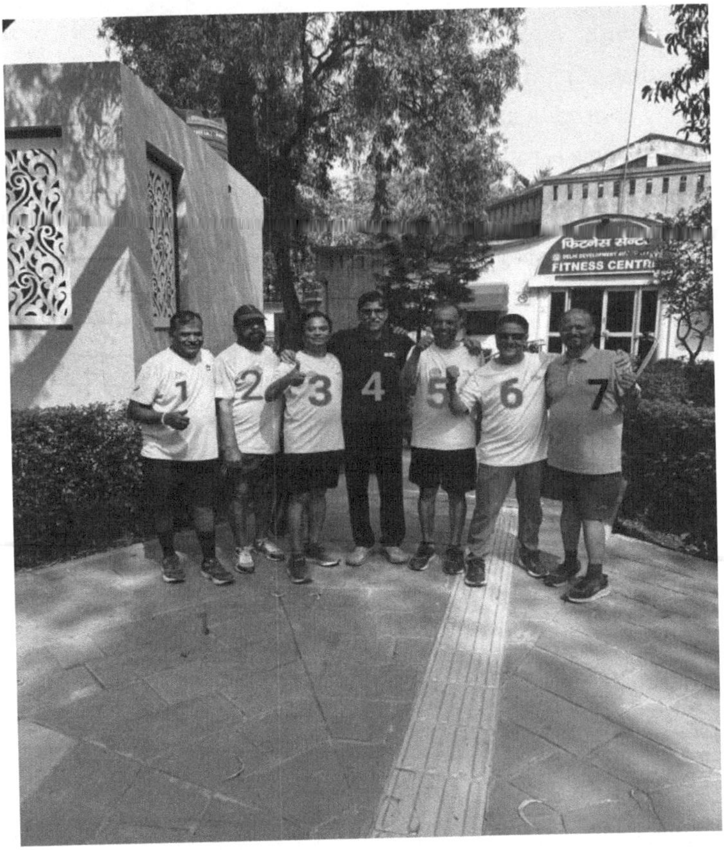

Sr.No	Name	Age in years	Marathon Km
1	Mr. B.S. Kapil	68	21 km
2	Mr. Dinesh Pande	65	10 km
3	Mr. Sanjaya Bhoi	61	21 km
4	Mr. Sanjeev Mahajan	56	21 km
5	Mr. Kailash Tewari	67	21 km
6	Mr. Bhushan Kaul	66	10 km
7	Mr. Girish Nigam	58	New student

Real inexpressible enjoyment

As I enjoy the daily running from the bottom of heart and share post running feeling to my friends in Chilla Sports Complex, Delhi (India) to motivate them to run and succeeded to make them participated in marathons at the age of more than 60 years. Above in chart are the names to whom I had motivated to participate in SMVD Katra marathon on 7Th April, 2023 and all of them touched finish line of marathon very successfully and they have proved that age is nothing but just a number and at any age with any body weight any one can start running. I myself enjoyed their success from the bottom of heart and which was really ecstatic and beyond the words and inexpressible.

When I touched the finished line in above marathon, of course it was moment of happiness but of average level because it was not my first time to touch the finish line.

But when my all motivated friends, all of them more than 60 years and were participating first time in half marathon (21)&10 km, successfully touched the finishing line, "O my God" there was nonverbal height of my ecstasy in my heart. They proved that age is just number and every seed has the capacity to become tree just by rejecting ephemeral comfort zone for very small period per day.

They are real my unsung hero in my life because they were very few in number amongst so many people to whom I tried to motivate.

My state of mind after touching finish line=1time = happiness= Ananad

My state of mind after touching the finish line by my motivated friends (6) =1x6=6times of my happiness=Ecstasy= Parmanand=Par+Ananad=Happiness due to others success

Hope they will remain in this zone forever and will be disciple of the Runligion.

"You are never too old to set another goal or to dream a new dream."

Inspired Zone

(List of some daily fuel (Kudos) suppliers out of 3,075 followers from all over the world to keep my spirit of running intact)

Kudos

ATHLETES YOU FOLLOW

Richard Bettesworth
Hayling Island

Ivair Basilio

Bhupendra Pandey
Ghaziabad, Vaishali

Ajay Dutta
Guwahati, ASSAM

Bejoy Jacob
Amritsar, Punjab

Glyn Pearson
Sharlston Common, England

Maria Leida! 👊🤪💯 Cada
Sabadell, Catalunya

Duong Tran
Surrey, England

Jayesh Mishra

Kudos

ATHLETES YOU FOLLOW

Shailesh Meshram

Tim France
Harrison, TN

Suresh Dwivedi
Jaipur, RAJASTHAN

James Riley 🚜🐝🌈
Rossendale, LANCASHIRE

Frederic Giovagnini 🇮🇹🏊🚴
Villeneuve-Loubet, Provence-Alp

RUPESH SINGH🇮🇳
Margao, Goa - INDIA

snegodoom 1967
Хабаровск, Хабаровский край

Zazou 🏊🚴🏃 Zerizazin

Prashant Tandon
New Delhi, Delhi

← Kudos

ATHLETES YOU FOLLOW

SR Dharmapal Fulzele : TIGE
Tiger City Cycling Association ,

Kane Travers
Chisholm, ACT

Robin Kapoor
Delhi, Delhi

Chandrashekhar Murthy
Bengaluru, Karnataka

Madan. M Trivedi
Noida, Uttar Pradesh

Dilip Dwivedi
Noida, UP

Priyaank Choubey
Bangalore, KARNATAKA

James Riley 🚜 🐝 🌈
Rossendale, LANCASHIRE

Harshad Kale
Mumbai/Chiplun, MAHARASHT

← Kudos

ATHLETES YOU FOLLOW

Anuj Gandhi
Delhi, Delhi

Crystal Hootman
Boulder, Colorado

Jitesh Thakkar
Nagpur, Maharashtra

Er. Uday Singh
Jaipur, Rajasthan

Jayesh Mishra

Mukesh Yadav
Delhi, DELHI

Sanjeev Menon
ಬೆಂಗಳೂರು, ಕರ್ನಾಟಕ

Varun Mahalle
Nagpur, MAHARASHTRA

Amit Kavimandan
AMRAVATI, Maharashtra

← Kudos

ATHLETES YOU FOLLOW

Prachi Kukde Tiger City Cyclin
Nagpur, MAHARASHTRA

Arvind Mandpe
Mumbai, Maharashtra

Craig Farham
Sedgefield, Western Cape

Ashok Singh

Robert Wróblewski
Kraków, małopolskie

Girish Balachandran
Thiruvananthapuram, KL

Megan Spicer
Coonabarabran, NSW

David Leedham 'V' (lovejoy)
Portelet,St.Brelade,, Jersey, Chanr

Manav Bhardwaj
Noida, Delhi

← Kudos

ATHLETES YOU FOLLOW

Sandeep Rattan
Simla, HP

Kailas Padawale
Pimpri-Chinchwad, Maharasht

Biswajit Bhattacharya
New Delhi, DL

Prem Rathod |AEC||ARHA
Ironman Pusad, MAHARASHT

Abhishek Bansal
Mumbai, Maharashtra

Ramesh G Gupta
Mumbai, Maharashtra

L R Pant

RUPESH SINGH
Margao, Goa - INDIA

Davy Dominic Moyalan
Thrissur, KL

← Kudos

ATHLETES YOU FOLLOW

Manpreet Grover 🇮🇳🇩🇰
Hvidovre

Sanjay Mahajan
Latur, MAHARASHTRA

Puji M.
Novara, Piemonte

Anuj Bansal 🇮🇳
Delhi

Dr. Somnath Babhale / RUN.
Kalyan, MAHARASHTRA

Bodhisattwa Dasgupta

Ayush Srivastava
Ghaziabad, UTTAR PRADESH

Vivek Ganjoo
New Delhi, Delhi

David M !
mt kisco, ny????????

← Kudos

ATHLETES YOU FOLLOW

SACHIT KOCHHAR
New Delhi, Delhi

Atishkumar Mali
Mumbai, Maharashtra

SR deepak parmar HRJ
JALANDHA, PUNJAB

MSG 문성기
한국, 부산시

Himanshu 🏃🚴🏊
Jaipur, RAJASTHAN

Suresh Dwivedi
Jaipur, RAJASTHAN

OTHER ATHLETES

Vanárts Faláringër
Santana Do Riacho, MG

Younus Mohammed

Mudit Agarwal
New Delhi, Delhi

← Kudos

ATHLETES YOU FOLLOW

Rajesh Sharma
New Delhi, DL

Dharmendra Srivastava
Greater Noida West, Uttar Prade:

Shekhar Balekar, TIGER CIT'
Nagpur, MAHARASHTRA

Shrikant Pandey
Gurgaon, HARYANA

Venky Vikram
New Delhi, DL

NoMore CloudyDays

SUDHIR SHARMA
Roorkee, Uttarakhand

Spring Social Paris Running &
paris

Nayan Kumar Das
Noida, UTTAR PRADESH

← Kudos

ATHLETES YOU FOLLOW

Alan Samuel
Bengaluru, Karnataka

Mahesh Nimhan 🚩🇮🇳🚩
Pune, Maharashtra

Ajay Dutta
Guwahati, ASSAM

Padmaparag Kelkar
Pune, MAHARASHTRA

Nishant Kaushik
Pune, Maharashtra

Glyn Pearson
Sharlston Common, England

vineet sharma
Noida, UTTAR PRADESH

Robin V
Noida, UTTAR PRADESH

Shashank D
Jhansi, Uttar Pradesh

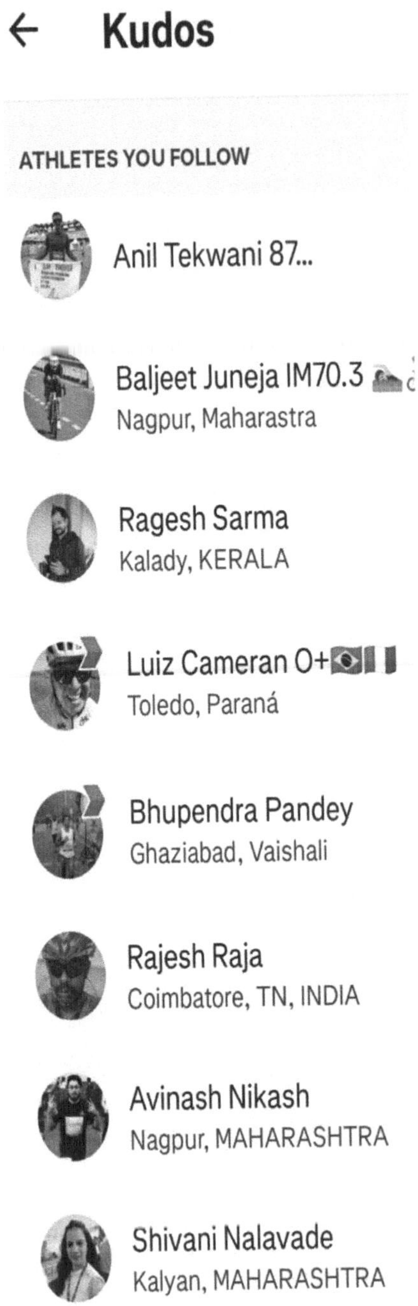
← Kudos
ATHLETES YOU FOLLOW
Anil Tekwani 87...
Baljeet Juneja IM70.3
Nagpur, Maharastra
Ragesh Sarma
Kalady, KERALA
Luiz Cameran O+
Toledo, Paraná
Bhupendra Pandey
Ghaziabad, Vaishali
Rajesh Raja
Coimbatore, TN, INDIA
Avinash Nikash
Nagpur, MAHARASHTRA
Shivani Nalavade
Kalyan, MAHARASHTRA

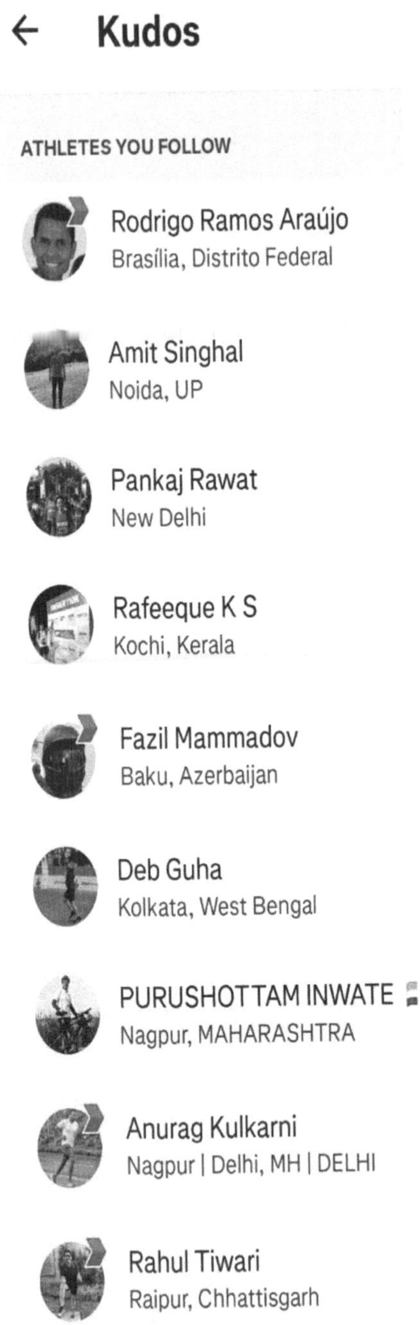
← Kudos
ATHLETES YOU FOLLOW
Rodrigo Ramos Araújo
Brasília, Distrito Federal
Amit Singhal
Noida, UP
Pankaj Rawat
New Delhi
Rafeeque K S
Kochi, Kerala
Fazil Mammadov
Baku, Azerbaijan
Deb Guha
Kolkata, West Bengal
PURUSHOTTAM INWATE
Nagpur, MAHARASHTRA
Anurag Kulkarni
Nagpur | Delhi, MH | DELHI
Rahul Tiwari
Raipur, Chhattisgarh

Kudos

ATHLETES YOU FOLLOW

Rajesh Raghuvanshi
New Delhi, DELHI

Anurag Vidhale
Nagpur, Maharashtra

Vijay Unde
Pimpri-Chinchwad, Maharashtr

Amarjit Giri
chandigarh, chandigarh

Barefoot Blond
Portsmouth, England

Aniruddha Sune
Dallas, Texas

Bejoy Jacob
Amritsar, Punjab

snegodoom 1967
Хабаровск, Хабаровский краі

Richard Bettesworth
Hayling Island

Kudos

ATHLETES YOU FOLLOW

Morne Gouws 🇿🇦
Akasia, Gauteng

Arjun Krishnakumar
Mumbai

Cesar Hernandez
Ocala, Florida

Zazou 🏊🚴🏃 Zerizazir

Alexander Bredikhin
Moscow, Russia

Chaitanya Deshpande
pune

Sanjib Nepram
Imphal, Manipur

Sorabh Babu
lucknow, Uttar Pradesh

Gurmeet Ahuja
New Delhi, Delhi

← **Kudos**

ATHLETES YOU FOLLOW

Mike F.
Lichtenstein/Sachsen, Sachsen

Bruce Semer
Greenwich, Connecticut

Stoyko Genchev
Sofia, Sofia-city

Suresh Dwivedi
Jaipur, RAJASTHAN

Bejoy Jacob
Amritsar, Punjab

Sachin Mendhe
Nagpur, Maharashtra

Simon Dunn
Liopetri, Famagusta

Satish Sharma 🏃 🚴
Pantnagar, Uttrakhand

Amit Singhal
Noida, UP

← **Kudos**

ATHLETES YOU FOLLOW

Sanjeev Menon
ಬೆಂಗಳೂರು, ಕರ್ನಾಟಕ

Usha Paliwal
Indrapuram, GZAI

snegodoom 1967
Хабаровск, Хабаровский край

Rajesh Raghuvanshi
New Delhi, DELHI

Ednilton Jesus da Silva
Salvador, Bahia

Umesh Patil
Kudus (Palghar), Thane, MAHARA

Amit Singhal
Noida, UP

Nitin Awalkar
Ichalkaranji, MAHARASHTRA

Crystal Hootman
Boulder, Colorado

Postface

Happiness index and runners percentage countrywide

Top 10 happiest countries in the world

Rank		Runners %
1.	Finland	43% (female)
2.	Denmark	
3.	Iceland	
4.	Sweden	
5.	Israel	
6.	Netherlands	
7.	Norway	
8.	Luxembourg	
9.	Switzerland	
10.	Australia	41%
126	India	**0.2 %**

India ranks 126th out of 143 countries,

Running data

2 Nov 2023 — the countries with the most female trail runners are: Finland - 43%; Australia - 41%; Canada - 39%. Running statistics by race distance. For a...

Physical activity, including running, is linked to happiness, and there is evidence that exercise can improve overall health and mental well-being:

- **Hormones**

Physical activity releases endorphins, serotonin, and dopamine, which can contribute to feelings of happiness and euphoria.

- **Stress**

Exercise can reduce stress levels by lowering cortisol.

- **Survey data**

A large survey of young adults in 24 countries found that those who were moderately or highly active had higher life satisfaction and happiness.

Er. Sunil Gajbhiye
January 19, 2025 at 5:22 AM · Mumbai, Maharashtra

Tata Mumbai Marathon Run

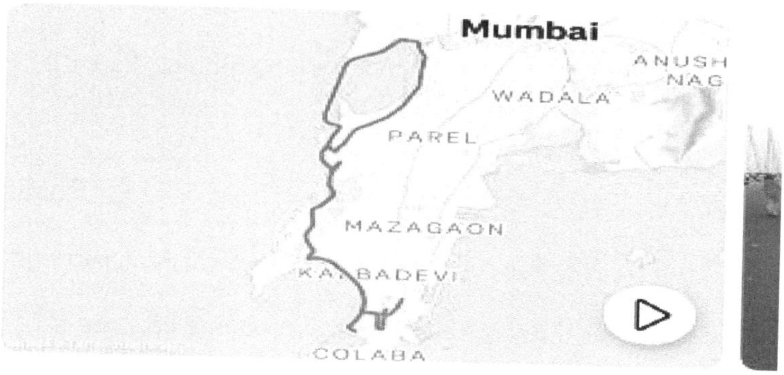

Distance	Avg Pace
42.83 km	**7:32 /km**
Moving Time	Elevation Gain
5:22:46	**108 m**
Calories	Avg Heart Rate
2,732 Cal	**151 bpm**

Above is data recorded by my watch Garmin 55.

TMM 2025:Bib number:2540, **14 meters above sea level**

SUNIL GAJBHIYE crossed the Finish at 10:56

Course time: 05:34:18

Pace: 07:56 min/km

Above is the data recorded by Marathon standstill watch in Mumbai, India

Differences are: Time recorded by Standstill watch-Time recorded by running watch

= 05:34:18-5:22:46=00:11:18

Before reading the book “THE ORDER OF TIME” (by CARLO ROVELLI) the thought over difference of covered distance in marathon was as under:-

Tata Mumbai Marathon on 19/01/2025

Start point A<..→B Finish point

42.2 Km Physical strait distance with no running, Pace= 0/ km,

Watch showed the distance

Start point A◄――――――――――――――――――――► C Finish point

42.83 Km running distance in watch, Avg. pace=7:32/km

Because of non-strait distance covered during running between start point and finish point.

$$AC\ (42.83) > AB\ (42.2)$$

$$AC-AB=42.83-42.2=0.63\ k$$

But after reading book “THE ORDER OF TIME” my thought over the difference of distance covered in marathon, IN WATCH got modified. As per book:-

The Slowing Down of Time

- Time passes faster in mountains than it does at sea level.
- *Speed Also Slows Down Time*

It means there are be three factors behind the difference of distance

- Non strait distance during running
- **Time passes faster in mountains than it does at sea level.**
- **Speed slows Down time**

For the third factor "**Speed slows down time**" I have compared the data from participated Tata Mumbai Marathon held on Jan 19, 2025 with data recorded by my running watch and found authenticity in second factor.

Running pace=7 minutes: 32 seconds /km= (7x60+32) =420+32

=452 second/ km

Extra time for 0.63km (AC-AB) =0.63x452=284.76 seconds= 284.76/60

=4:76 minutes (approx.)

Tata Mumbai marathon **at 14 meters above sea level**

But as per watch extra time=11:18

Therefore effect of Order of time =11:18-4:76=6:02

Because speed slows down time, here speed slows down time by

6 minutes: 02 seconds (approx.) Near sea level

Resultant Effect of Order of Time 6:02

Height 14 meters

Above

Sea level

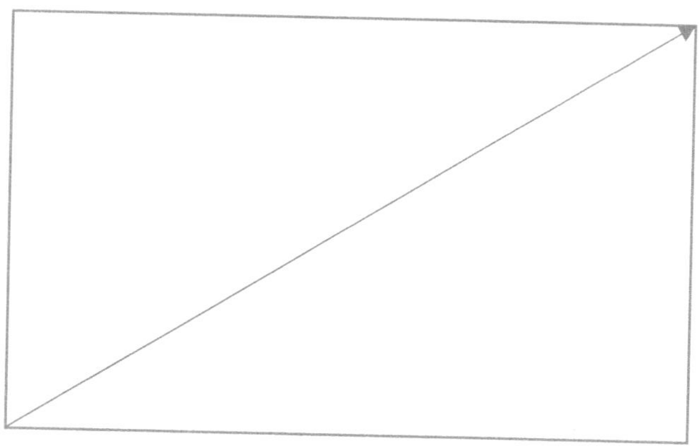

Pace 7:32/km=Speed 7.7 kmph

Slower speed than marathon in Delhi because of elevation gain of 108 meters at lower height above sea level is exhibiting significant difference of time of 6:02 minutes because of law of ORDER OF TIME.

Speed slows down time and time passes faster in near the mountain area

Slow speed (7.7kmph) fasts up time⟶

Time passes slower near sea level (14 meters) ⟶

Second practical example is Apollo New Delhi Marathon on February 23, 2025 for Second factor:-

Time passes faster in mountains than it does at sea level.

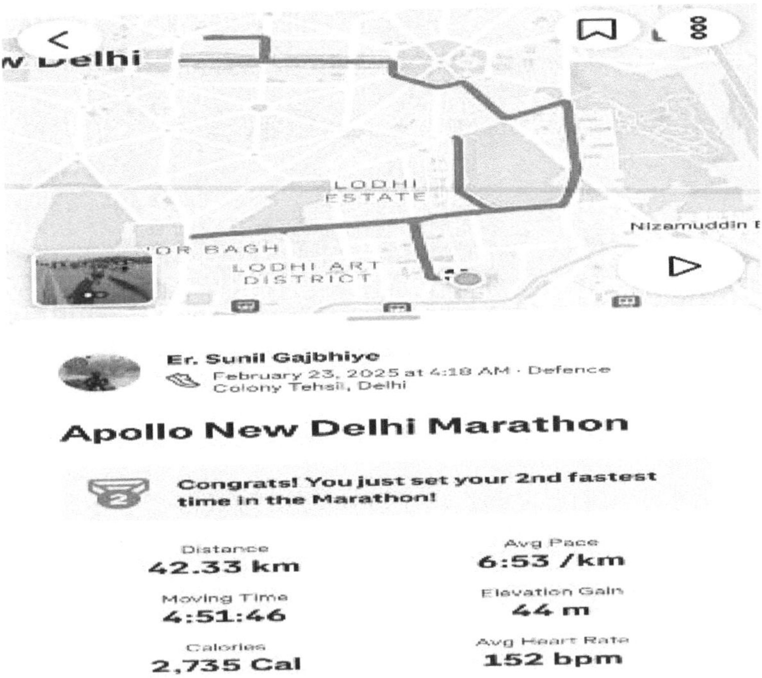

Above is data recorded by my watch Garmin 55.

Apollo Tyres New Delhi: **216 meters above sea level**

SUNIL GAJBHIYE crossed the Finish at 09:14

Course time: 04:56:17

Pace: 07:02 min/km

Above is the data recorded by Marathon standstill watch

Differences are: Time recorded by Standstill watch-Time recorded by moving watch

Time difference =4:56:17-4:51:46=00:04:31

Distance difference=42.33-42.2=0.13 km

Before reading the book "THE ORDER OF TIME" (by CARLO ROVELLI) the thought over difference of covered distance in marathon was as under:-

Apollo New Delhi Marathon on 23/02/2025

Start point A.. B Finish point

42.2 Km Physical strait distance with no running, Pace= 0/ km,

Watch showed the distance

Start point A ←——————————————→ C Finish point

42.33 km running distance in watch, pace=6:53/km

Distance difference = AC-AB= =42.33-42.2=0.13km

Running pace=6 minutes: 53 seconds /km= (6x60+53)=360+53

=413 second/ km

Extra time for 0.13km=0.13x413=284.76 seconds= 284.76/60

=4.746 minutes (approx.) =4:44(approx.)

But as per watch extra time=04:31

Therefore effect of" Order of time" = 04:31-4:44= (0:13) second.

Resultant Effect of Order of Time (0.13) seconds

Delhi marathon

Height at 216

Meters above

Sea level

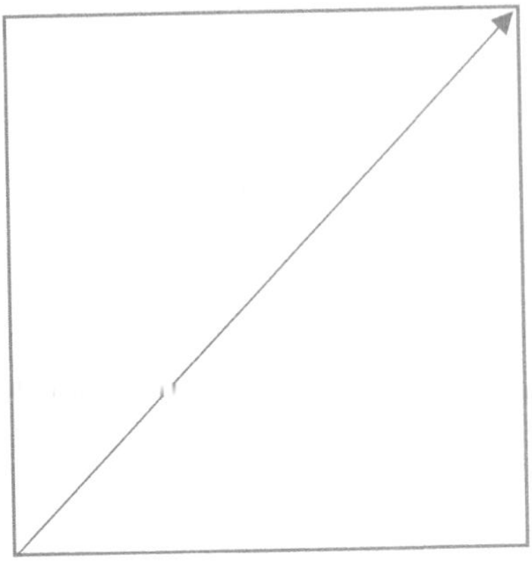

Pace 6:53/km= Speed 9.1 kmph

Higher speed at more height above sea level exhibiting difference of time of only (0:13) second and thus mostly **neutralize** the effect of each other because of following two laws of ORDER OF TIME.

1. Speed slows down time and
2. Time passes faster in near the mountain area

Tata Mumbai Marathon Running pace-**7:32/km** with elevation gain 108 m **at14 meters above sea level**

Apollo New Delhi marathon running pace- **6:53/km** with elevation gain 44 m **at 216 meters above sea level**

Time passes faster in mountains than it does at sea level (Marathon in Delhi at 216 meters above sea level).

Speed slows down time (marathon In Mumbai at 14 meters above sea level)

So authenticity of above two law during running at near sea level (Mumbai) and above sea level (Delhi) is categorically visible.

For the law "speed slow down the time" I have done practical running in Chilla Sport omplex Delhi, India, to test it.

First experiment on March 29th,2025 in Chilla Sport Complex Delhi India

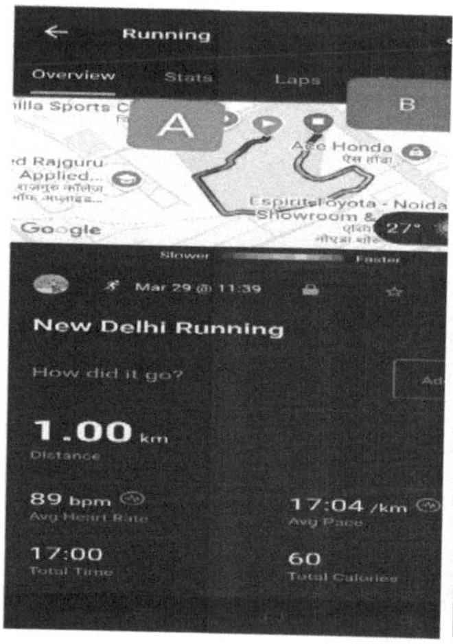

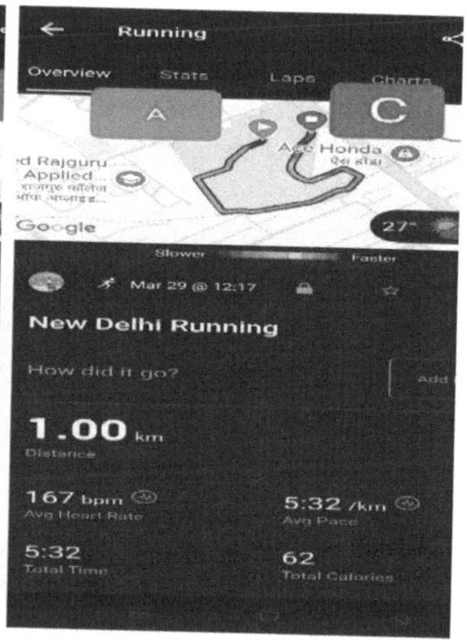

AB(at 17:04/km slower speed)<AC(at 5:32/Km higher speed)

A...B

at 17:04/km slower speed (Distance=1Km in watch)

A...C

at 5:32/Km higher speed (Distance=1Km,in watch)

AC-AB=BC(difference in distance=0.03Km)

B.................................C

0.03 Km at 19:53/km

Higher speed slow down the time by BC distance (0.03Km) running time=0:31(approx.) at 19:53/Km.

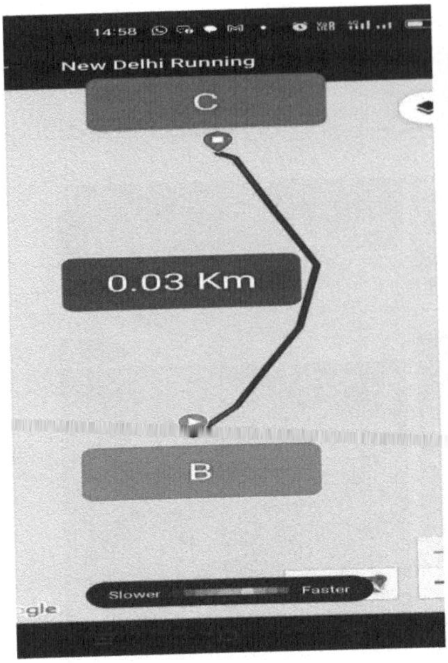
14:58
New Delhi Running
C
0.03 Km
B
Slower
Faster

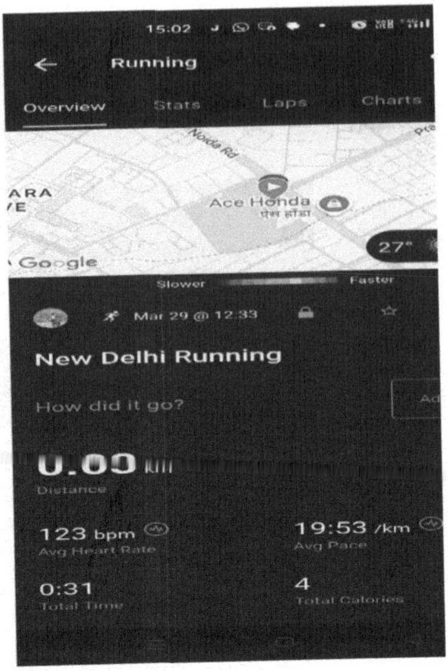
15:02
Running
Overview
Stats
Laps
Charts
Noida Rd
Ace Honda
27°
Slower
Faster
Mar 29 @ 12:33
New Delhi Running
How did it go?
Distance
123 bpm
Avg Heart Rate
19:53 /km
Avg Pace
0:31
Total Time
4
Total Calories

Second experiment in Chilla Sport complex Delhi, India on May15th,2-25

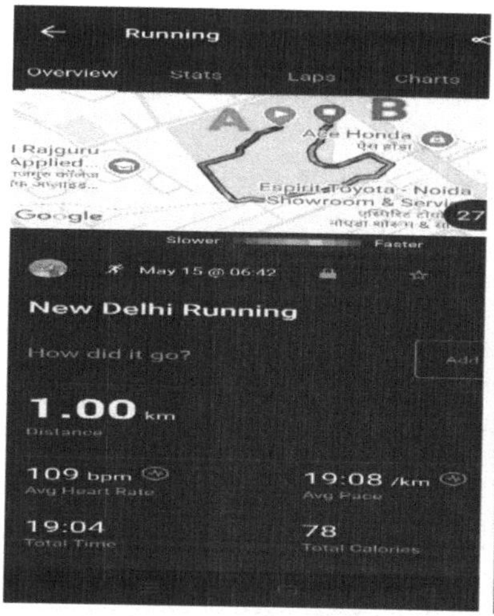

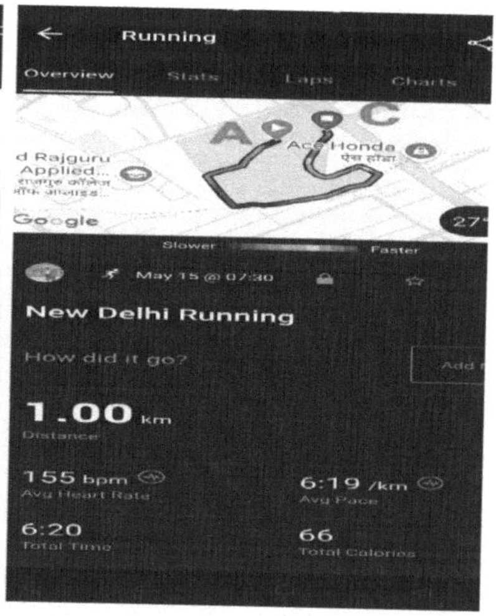

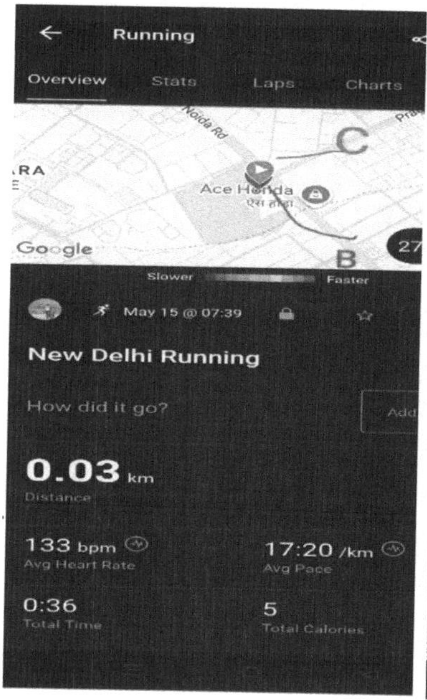

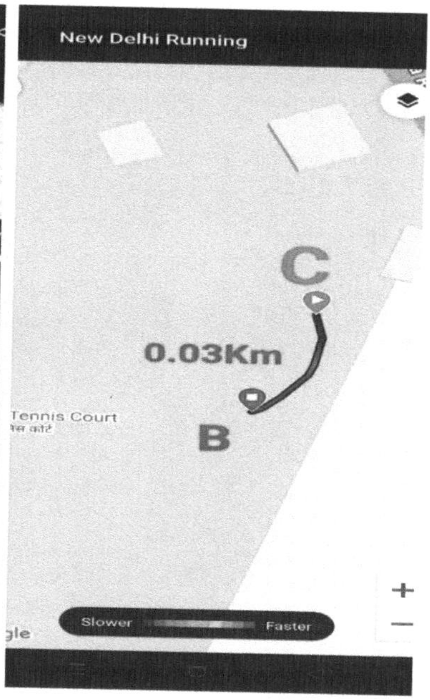

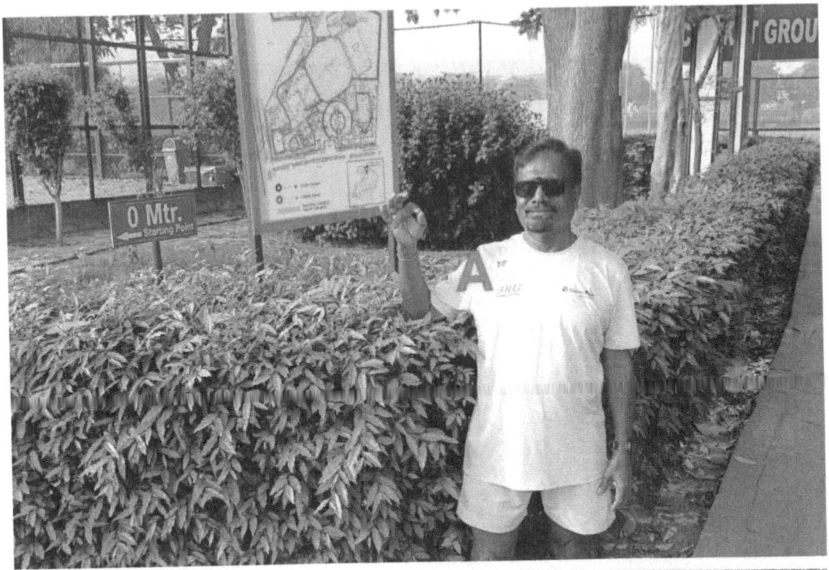
0 Mtr.
Starting Point
A

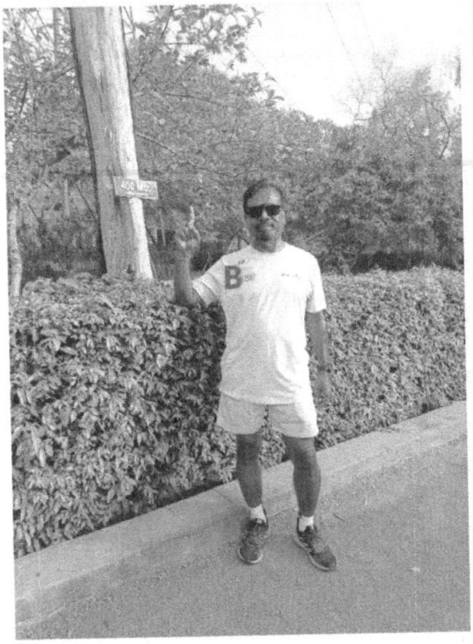
B

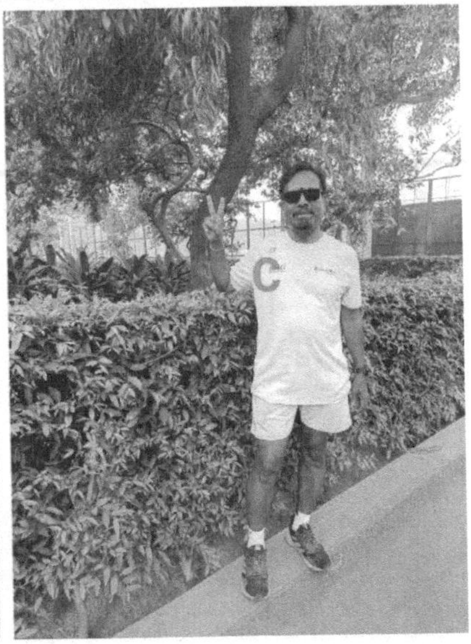
C

AB (at 19:08/km slower speed)<AC(at 6:19/Km higher speed)

A..B

at 19:08/km slower speed (Distance=1Km in watch)

A..C

at 6:19/Km higher speed (Distance=1Km,in watch)

AC-AB=BC=Difference in distance=0.03Km

B..................................C

=0.03Km

Higher speed slow down the time by BC distance (0.03Km) running time=0:36(approx.) at 17:20/Km.

Gist of experiment:-

AC> AB, by BC=0.03KM=30 meters because, speed slow down the time and hence Runners of same age are younger than non-runners because of the "THE ORDER OF TIME', as per author,

The one who moves ages less quickly, his watch marks less time passing; he has a less time in which to think; the plant he is carrying takes longer to germinate, and so on. For everything that moves, time passes more slowly.

A moving object therefore experience a shorter duration than a stationary one: a watch marks fewer seconds, a plant grows more slowly, a young man dreams less. For moving object time contracts.

Therefore, in case of runner and non-runner at the age of 60 years, runner ages less quickly and hence he looks younger than non-runner. Running increases average life span.

10:34

(Er.Sunil Gajbhiye

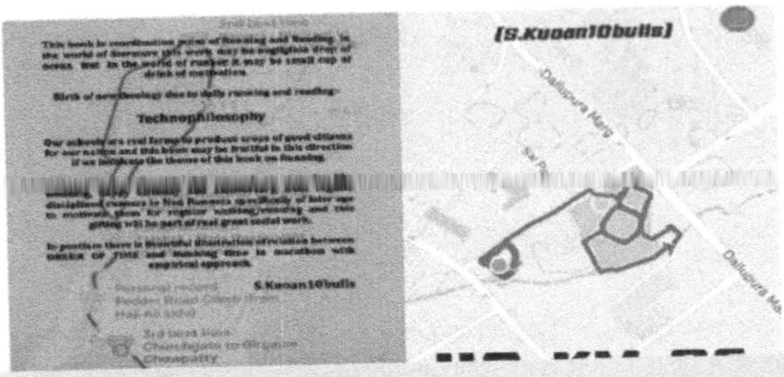

W book publishing.docx

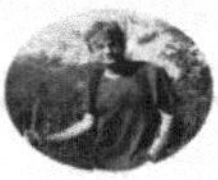

carlo rovelli Yesterday

to me

nice! thanks!
c

Show quoted text

--

Reply

MBA (management of body ability) Health Dairy

Name:-

Age:-

Weight before starting run (A) = _____

Targeted weight as per BMI (B) = ______

Extra burden on heart as per BMI (A-B) = __________

Sr.No.	Date	Morning Bed leaving Time	Run start time	Distance KM	Gear	Extra Burden as per BMI(A-B) Kg
1						
2						
3						
4						
5						
6						
7						
8						
9						
10						
11						
12						
13						
14						
15						
16						
17						
18						
19						
20						
21						
22						
23						
24						
25						
26						
27						
28						
29						
30						
31						

Sr.No.	Date	Morning Bed leaving Time	Run start time	Distance KM	Gear	Extra Burden as per BMI(A-B) Kg
1						
2						
3						
4						
5						
6						
7						
8						
9						
10						
11						
12						
13						
14						
15						
16						
17						
18						
19						
20						
21						
22						
23						
24						
25						
26						
27						
28						
29						
30						
31						

Sr.No.	Date	Morning Bed leaving Time	Run start time	Distance KM	Gear	Extra Burden as per BMI(A-B) Kg
1						
2						
3						
4						
5						
6						
7						
8						
9						
10						
11						
12						
13						
14						
15						
16						
17						
18						
19						
20						
21						
22						
23						
24						
25						
26						
27						
28						
29						
30						
31						

Sr.No.	Date	Morning Bed leaving Time	Run start time	Distance KM	Gear	Extra Burden as per BMI(A-B) Kg
1						
2						
3						
4						
5						
6						
7						
8						
9						
10						
11						
12						
13						
14						
15						
16						
17						
18						
19						
20						
21						
22						
23						
24						
25						
26						
27						
28						
29						
30						
31						

This is the first series of 42 episodes of *Technophiloshophy on running*

The second series of 33 episodes of *Technophilosophy on running* "33 Km of Runligion" is in womb.

S.Kuoanɪobulls

(Er. Sunil Gajbhiye)

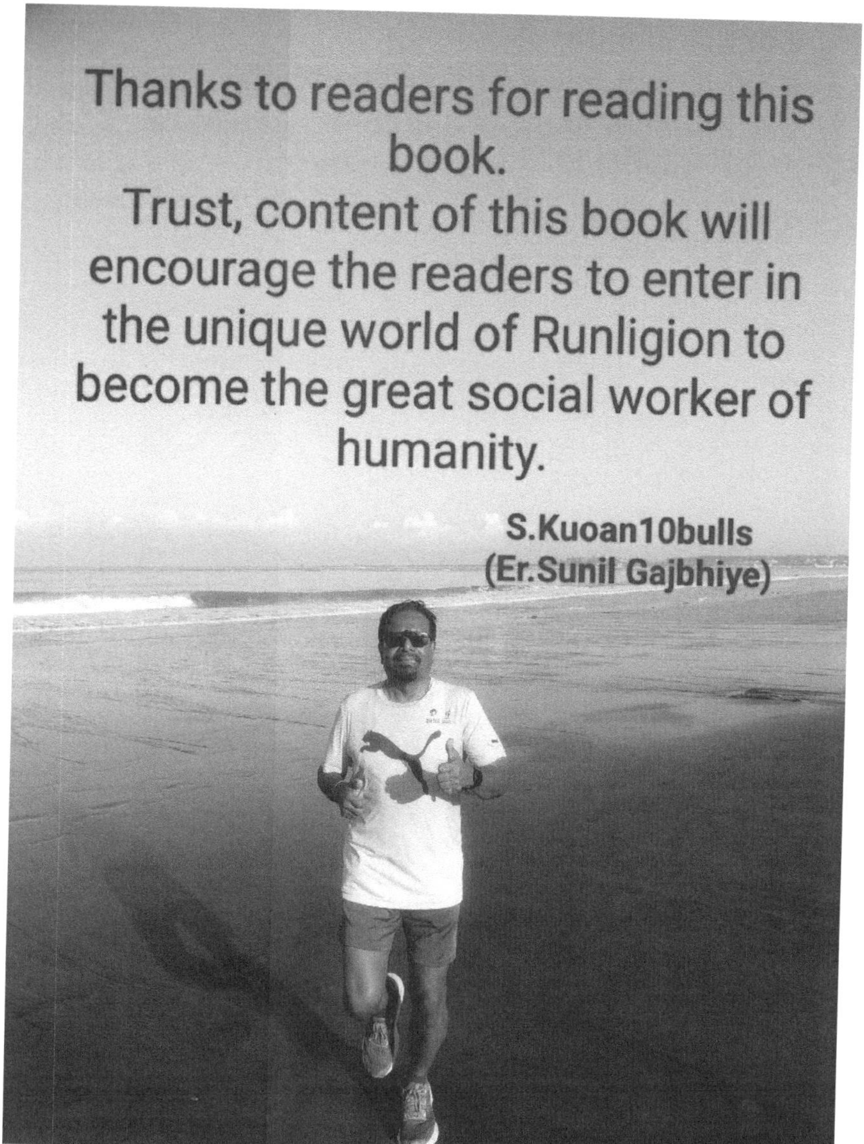
Thanks to readers for reading this book.
Trust, content of this book will encourage the readers to enter in the unique world of Runligion to become the great social worker of humanity.
S.Kuoan10bulls
(Er.Sunil Gajbhiye)